SASHA DEOL

THE 7 PILLARS
• OF •
WELLNESS

A SIMPLE GUIDE TO GET YOUR
LIFE BACK ON TRACK

San Francisco, CA

ISBN: 978-1-7343892-2-7 (Paperback)
ISBN: 978-1-7343892-0-3 (Hardcover)
ISBN: 978-1-7343892-1-0 (eBook)

Library of Congress Control Number: 2019919846

The intent of the author is to offer general information to assist you in your quest for being a better version of yourself. The author and publisher assume no responsibility for your actions, consequences, loss or damage of any type, or adverse effects arising from any use or application of any content herein. The author does not claim or guarantee any benefits, healing, cure or any results in any way and shall not be liable or responsible for use of content application from this publication. All efforts have been made to assure the accuracy of the information contained in this book as of the date of publication.

First edition April 2020

www.the7pillarsofwellness.com

San Francisco, CA

TABLE OF CONTENTS

The 7 Pillars of Wellness: Introduction

Since this guide views your health holistically, it's necessary to analyze various aspects of your life and make sure they are harmonious. What does "holistic" even mean? Having a holistic view means looking at multiple areas as they relate to a whole, in this case, your body. There is rarely one single factor that can make or break your health. You need to look deeper into your existence to figure out what's really going on. When taking the holistic approach to improve your health, you must look at *everything* when it comes to achieving your optimal health. In medicine, this means searching for root causes, instead of treating symptoms. When taking a holistic approach to life, you acknowledge different parts of your life are important when it comes to your *whole* life.

Consider the following as the 7 Pillars of Wellness: nutrition, social, emotional, mental, spiritual, physical and integrity. When re-evaluating your life, carefully address each of these things and think about how you can improve them. The order of the 7 Pillars is not of importance, they must all be incorporated into your life. As you read, you may notice there are overlapping themes within this book. For example, stress management can be addressed under multiple pillars, such as spiritual and emotional, as well as the physical Pillar of Wellness. This is because they each play an important role contributing to your life as a whole. You will see this as you read through each section and begin to make practical, easy changes in your life. I've done plenty of research over the years and discovered some things that can transform your life, making it better than ever.

I was inspired to write this book to show you how to incorporate easy, practical tips and tricks into your everyday life to improve it. I invested quite some time at my alma mater learning about the science of animals, humans and the Earth. Initially, I had no idea what I would do with this knowledge, only to later realize that it all made sense. Over time, conversation around cancer and disease became a recurring theme, along with unhappiness, depression, sickness and discontentment amongst people I interacted with. I wanted to know why. One common denominator I observed was high stress, poor diet and a not-so-great lifestyle.

I started looking back at what I had studied. The animals I worked with over the years were fed diets comprising of processed corn and grain, but their stomachs were designed to digest unprocessed products that came directly from the Earth, such as grass. The processed foods cause the animals to grow at a faster rate than animals fed a natural diet. Because the animals cannot digest these diets properly, hormones and antibiotics are pumped into the animals to prevent illness. Eventually, the animals are slaughtered and consumed by humans. It all comes full circle when you learn a bad diet can lead to health problems in humans. This is but one of many puzzles I pieced together in the journey to help others prevent illness and reach their full potential of health and happiness. If health and happiness pique your interest, you will benefit from integrating the things you learn in this book into your life.

Ultimately, it comes down to two things: you must be better and things are only as hard as you make them. Remember that. Look at the bigger picture—your problems generally never root from one single thing. Whether your goals are to lose weight, gain strength or maintain health, fixing your diet, exercising and managing stress will improve your life overall.

Lucky for you, I've done the boring research, read the scientific journals and collected information to create a guide of applicable tips you can start using right away! You deserve to have a healthy, beautiful body and life. You deserve to be happy. You deserve to live the most vibrant life you can and be the best version of yourself. Let's begin learning about the 7 Pillars of Wellness.

Pillar I:
Nutrition

There are so many basic life skills many of us were never taught in school: how to do taxes, mental health management, self-defense, the art of balance, how to eat healthy, the list goes on. Sure, I remember an optional health education elective in high school where teachers shelled out the standard, archaic food pyramid and explained the "importance" of drinking milk (one of the many things that have been proven wrong). The food pyramid has since been replaced with some plate diagram sponsored by powerful industry players pushing their products—meat, dairy, sugar, soda... you catch my drift.

Over time, I have changed my diet significantly, as it is always a work in progress. There are great days and weeks, just as there are setbacks and failures. The one thing that stays consistent is that I keep pushing forward. You should, too. I believe the key to maintaining a wholesome diet is balance and practice. As cliché as it might sound, it's true and shall forever remain so. We are all human and no one is perfect. Striving for constant perfection only results in going down a rabbit hole of stress paired with unrealistic expectations and standards. Accept that there will be times when you "fall off" and have something that's not on your diet, whether it's due to lack of self-control or out of necessity.

Fret not, for it's not the end of the world. **Keep pushing forward**. The problem arises when you mess up that one time and give up completely. When tempted or in doubt, remind yourself of your end goal: looking, feeling and being overall fabulous! Make a small investment for your well-being now and continually reap the benefits for the rest of your life. It does not matter how old or young you are because it's never too late to start. We all deserve to feel amazing, confident and full of life!

Take a little time to prepare

One of the keys to success is preparation. As the saying goes, "Success happens when preparation meets opportunity." Sure, you can tell yourself "I don't have time!" but guess what? Not many of us "have" time. You need to *make* time. Sit down and take 30 minutes out of the 10,080 minutes (168 hours!) you have in a week to jot down a basic meal plan. Write down what you're going to eat for the week and make a grocery list. If you're feeling extra ambitious, plan out two weeks' worth of meal plans. Doing this simple task will cut out the frustrating questions we all experience from time to time:

"What is there to eat?"

"What am I going to eat?"

"What should I eat?"

I, for one, hate meal prepping and being in the kitchen, slaving over a stove or breaking my back doing dishes. It's neither my forte, nor my favorite thing to do, hence the words I choose to describe the task. That being said, I have been working on reframing the whole "slaving over a stove" and "breaking my back doing dishes" mentality to avoid having such a negative attitude towards the meal-prep process. I've discovered ways around the dread by reminding myself things are only as hard as you make them, and cooking up a more enjoyable experience by listening to an audiobook or enlisting someone to join me. Plus, it's all about streamlining the process, especially if you're lazy, like me. A simple strategy I have come up with is:

1. Plan
2. Purchase
3. Prep

Plan out your diet for the week by making a list of ingredients you need to buy for recipes and meals, then go purchase what you need and prepare what you can. I try to keep things minimal—for example, I'll cut down on meal prep time by getting easy fruit you can wash, grab and go, like apples and bananas. In order to minimize dishes, I have invested in an Instant Pot. An Instant Pot works wonders for me because you can "set it and forget it." Plus, you need less cookware in your kitchen since it has so many capabilities, ranging from cooking a side of rice to full meals such as Indian Chana Masala. If you don't know what to eat, find some recipes online to get started or look up basic meal plan ideas for the diet of your choice (I would highly recommend plant-based, or at least vegetarian). Then, it's time to shop and prep.

Once you've got your ingredients, it's time to get the ball rolling in the kitchen. Things should move quickly since you're about halfway through the process at this point. It just takes a little bit of time to get the hang of things, retrain yourself and reframe your views. You can't go in with the mindset that you hate meal prep, otherwise the process will feel as if it's dragging on. It's better to neutralize the negative feelings rather than agonize over what you're doing. I like to try to get into a flow state when I'm meal prepping in order to get done with it as soon as possible.

Get into a flow state of mind

A flow state is when you are completely immersed in whatever it is you are doing. You lose track of time and forget everything else. Often, people are in a flow state when they are doing something they absolutely love. You can motivate yourself to get through any task such as meal prepping by striving to reach a state of flow. A bonus is enhanced performance and getting through the task more efficiently while being in a better state of mind.[1]

My plan-purchase-prep technique is designed so you can achieve a flow state of mind. It has a specific goal and plan of action. If you want to try to achieve a flow state of mind, in addition to having a specific goal and plan of action, creating an element of challenge and trying to stretch your current skill level can help. Ideally, the activity should be something you enjoy or are passionate about.[2] So, when it comes to meal prep:

- Your passion can root from working on improving your body
- The specific goal is to get the meal prep done, with plan of action being plan, purchase, prep
- Challenge yourself by trying new recipes or foods
- Stretch your current skill set by trying to become more efficient each time

See, doesn't this all seem elementary now? I'm hoping with the rest of the information in this guide, I can equip you with the right tools to start thriving in life imme-diately. Read on.

Effortless, nutritious calories

While you're in the planning phase of meal prep, especially when you are starting out, you may feel like it's hard to come up with ideas on what to eat and what to have for snacks. Go easy on yourself and keep it simple! The best part about eating healthy is that it's so basic that it will become nearly effortless over time. Consider the following scenarios:

It's breakfast time: have a banana. One serving of fruit done! Pair it with something easy, like a peach, apple, pear. Two servings of fruit done first thing in the morning! Need some caffeine? Have some green tea. One glass of water, some antioxidants, plus a little boost—done! Side note: substantial research shows a correlation between the consumption of green tea and both weight and fat loss.[3-5]

Need some snacks between meals? Choose some whole fruit, carrots and cucumbers since they are fresh and light, along with some homemade trail mix. If you must have something sweet, instead of a sugary, processed granola bar, have some nuts and dark chocolate. It will be easier on your stomach and wallet. Keep these kinds of snacks readily available, in your backpack or purse so that you can avoid going off your diet in times of hunger crisis!

For lunches and dinners, pre-cut some salad so it's ready to go with your lunches and dinners to get more servings of leafy greens. If you are a fan of bean and rice dishes, make some rice for the next couple days along with different kinds of beans. An Instant Pot is great for this, but if you don't have one, you can always use a rice cooker or the stove. Once you practice a bit and start learning to get into a state of flow with your meal prep, you will be on the road to success.

I've put together some lists and charts of healthy food info at the end of this section and in the appendix to help with your meal planning. Bookmark it with a sticky note so you can quickly reference it as needed.

Practice mindful eating

Now that the food-prepping situation has been addressed, let's discuss the process of eating. This sounds very rudimentary, but you'd be surprised by the impact small things have on your overall well-being. Without realizing it, you can fall into the habit of swallowing your food before fully chewing it, especially when you take too big or too small of bites. The first time chewing even came to my mind was when I went to a wellness spa for a deep-tissue massage. They offered colonic hydrotherapy, so, out of curiosity, I asked what that was. After a long discussion about the procedure and benefits of colonic therapy, I learned one thing: when you don't chew your food properly, you end up wasting nutrients and risk developing digestive issues. If you're interested in learning more about the whole chewing thing, read on. If not, I took the liberty of conducting some research and all you really need to know is make sure to chew your food thoroughly to get the maximum nutritional value out of it; focus on chewing several times, which will make you eat slower, potentially improve digestion, reduce how much you eat and enhance the enjoyability of your meal.[2, 6-8] Now, for the details...

Digestion starts with your teeth and saliva when you break food down into smaller pieces, making it easier to digest and allowing the greatest amount of nutrient extraction for your body. One study I've come across states it's best to chew food approximately 32 times before swallowing.[9] This can definitely vary; if you're chewing soft and water-filled food, it won't require as much work but if you are chewing a mouthful of food that's harder to chew, for instance, nuts or meat, it may require up to 40 chews.[8-10] As a rule of thumb, chew until the food loses its texture. Curious? Try counting how many chews it takes to break down whatever you're eating. Between 32 and 40 bites? More or less?

Another downside of eating too fast and not chewing enough is that you are likely to eat more food. By chewing several times, at a slower pace, you will decrease your caloric intake (which is good, especially for weight loss). Research suggests those who eat slower consume signify-cantly less food, feel fuller than those who eat faster and snack less later in the day.[7, 11] Another study I examined found that chewing almonds 25-40 times before swallow-ing both suppressed hunger and increased the ability to absorb nutrients.[10] Moral of the story: don't rush when it comes to eating.

In theory, this could mean if you're eating healthy food, chew it thoroughly to maximize the benefits from the nutrient-rich foods, but, on the other hand, if you're eating unhealthy food, chew it less so your body doesn't absorb it as much, or better yet, don't eat it at all. But hey, this is my own theory; use at your own discretion! However, there are disadvantages when you choose not to chew properly, including[12]:

- Bloating
- Diarrhea
- Heartburn
- Acid reflux
- Cramps
- Nausea
- Headaches
- Skin problems
- Irritability
- Malnutrition
- Indigestion
- Gas

There you have it, a whole section on something as simple as chewing. Thought it would be a good idea to touch on it since, as mentioned earlier, it can be something easily forgotten and unlearned. The goal is to help you become aware of and improve your eating habits to achieve your optimal health.

Can't stop overeating?

Do you struggle with self-control when it comes to food and cravings? Do you eat until you're stuffed and bloated? Or perhaps you partake in emotional eating when under stress? We all have our struggles, and you're not alone in this one. There are plenty of ways to stop these uncomfortable and unhealthy habits; you just need to retrain yourself.

One of the most effective techniques I use is limiting accessibility to unhealthy foods. My weaknesses include sweets and chocolates, so I avoid buying them because I can rarely eat just one at a time. If I have them at home, I know I'll eat the junk food until it's all gone and wake up the next day with pimples. However, if they're not readily available, it makes it harder for me to get up at midnight and waltz into the kitchen for a little midnight chocolate nightcap. Know your weaknesses and have nutritious, alternative choices ready to snack on to avoid setbacks in your diet. Keep in mind, don't be *too* strict and deprive yourself of your absolute favorites from time to time—this can lead to binge eating when you get your hands on the foods you crave. Allow yourself some rewards in small amounts throughout the week.

While at the table, put away distractions and enjoy some fiber-rich veggies before a main dish. Avoid sitting in front of the TV or being on your phone or computer while you are eating. You will likely lose track of how much you are really eating and won't be mindful, eating more than a sufficient proportion.[13, 14] When it comes to proper serving sizes, never eat straight out of the package, instead, measure out the right serving size and limit yourself to that. Try using smaller dishes and plates so you eat less. Additionally, starting off your meal with non-starchy veggies such as fresh greens, broccoli or a light salad will not only prep your stomach for the meal and get a serving of veggies in, it will also help you feel full and make you less likely to overeat.[15, 16] Another habit that can make all the difference is to avoid skipping meals and eat fiber-rich foods (beans, vegetables, fruits, oats). Eating balanced meals throughout the day will help prevent overeating later on in the day and you will feel satisfied longer with fiber-rich foods.[16-20]

Reduce binge eating by practicing mindful eating and, if possible, surround yourself with people that have healthy eating habits. These two factors can greatly help break the habit of overindulgence. Being aware of your thoughts and senses while eating can reduce binge eating, over-eating and emotional eating.[13, 14, 19, 21-23] Make sure you properly chew your food since that will help you eat slower and maximize the nutrients you can get from your meals.[10, 12] Furthermore, extensive research on dining companions suggests your eating habits are greatly influenced by the people with whom you eat.[22] If you have the luxury of dining with someone who is also into healthy eating, you will likely be more inclined to order healthier options, and vice versa when your partner does. Plus, people generally tend to eat proportions similar to those of the people around them.[21, 22]

Eating healthy fats, protein and fiber-rich foods and foods that keep your blood sugar levels constant can prevent overeating. Healthy fats and protein-rich meals will keep you full and decrease the desire to eat until you can't anymore. Having a good balance of protein, fat and carbohydrates in your meals can significantly aid in combating cravings and hunger. While planning out your meals, you want to make sure you're not having large portions of foods that will make your blood sugar levels spike and sink like the stock market. It is vital to stabilize your blood sugar levels, as rapid blood sugar fluctuations promote hunger and may lead to overeating.[16, 17] So instead of eating white bread, sugary cookies and candy or other foods with high glycemic indices, choose foods like beans, oats, quinoa and brown rice to avoid rapid fluctuations in blood sugar levels.

Do you overindulge when it comes to drinking, having more than two drinks in a sitting? Pay special attention if you enjoy adult beverages. Hate to break it to you, but as you probably know, consuming alcohol isn't conducive to performing at your best. Alcohol plays a role in overeating, as it clouds your judgment and stimulates your appetite. In fact, several studies indicate having multiple drinks in one sitting may lead to overeating. If you feel you cannot forgo alcohol entirely, try to stick to one or two drinks to start and drink them very slowly.[24, 25] Yes, we live in a time where drinking excessively is normalized, but you have nothing to prove to anyone but yourself. If you want to drink, drink in moderation. If you can go without drinking at all, more power to you; you'll feel much better than everyone else the next morning.

Last, but not least, you need to have the right mindset. Remember your end goal while eating and instead of going on a fad diet that will likely fizzle out, try having more balanced meals and enjoy what you're eating. Have short and long-term goals when it comes to your eating habits and write them down and refer to them frequently. For instance, if you are overwhelmed with this whole process, you can start by having at least 3 carrots a day and move up to having 3 servings of vegetables daily. Look deeper and address *why* you overeat—is it boredom, depression, lack of self-control? If necessary, seek help from a professional. **The power to change rests in your hands—strive to be the best version of yourself**. Be patient while breaking your old habits and replacing them with these healthier, positive ones. It can take time to experience changes, but in the end, it will be worth it. Do it for yourself.

See what works for you

Once you start a new diet, you may experience some changes nearly immediately, or it may take more time. It takes approximately six to eight weeks to see significant changes when you start a new diet, medication, workout plan or habit. There are so many different diets out there—keto, paleo, vegan, see-food diet, you name it. Over time, the same diets often get renamed, without any new benefits. I've experimented with various diets over the years and settled on eating mostly whole, plant-based foods. I feel a plant-based diet is excellent for not only losing weight but improving your overall health as well. I did not grow up vegetarian or eating a very healthy diet, but after my father's first heart attack, our family changed our eating habits drastically to what was, at the time, recommended for heart patients. Looking back, I think the diet we were advised to adopt was not the best. I wish the general public, as well as physicians, were better informed on how to manage health problems and prevent illnesses.

A while back, I was in a Toastmaster's group where one of the members had suffered from a heart attack. He was in his mid-40s, very active and athletic, had a decent diet and drank in moderation. Being a family man, he wanted to be the best father to his children he could and be around for them as long as possible. His doctor told him he needed to make extreme lifestyle changes in order to live a long, fruitful life after his heart attack. He switched from the standard American diet to a plant-based diet, quit drinking, learned to manage his stress and continued to exercise regularly. This guy said he felt better than ever after making some necessary lifestyle changes. Following a speech about his experience, I discussed my father's health concerns with him. He recommended a book by Caldwell Esselstyn, *Prevent and Reverse Heart Disease*, which I found fascinating. After reading it and learning about the scientific research that has proven you can reverse and heal serious illnesses by changing your diet, I decided to give the plant-based diet a shot, hoping my father would join me.

It took a bit of time to adjust at first, but I tried my best to make it exciting and have an enthusiastic approach. When friends and family learned that I had become vege-tarian or plant-based, they became very concerned with where I got my protein from, eventually making me question if I was getting enough or if the protein was good enough. As it turns out, we've been misled to believe we need way more protein than we actually do. And honestly, it's not as hard as you may think it is to get all the nutrients you need daily on a plant-based diet. Let's address the protein problem, since that's normally everyone's first question when they hear about non-meat diets.

The protein problem

Of the three macronutrients (carbohydrates, protein, fat) we need, protein is likely the most discussed when it comes to diet. Protein is made up of 20 different amino acids, compromised of nine essential amino acids and eleven non-essential amino acids. Non-essential amino acids are naturally synthesized by our body. We need to get the remaining nine essential amino acids from food. These essential amino acids can be found in plants. Animals get their protein directly or indirectly through the food chain from plants. A common misconception is that plant-based proteins are of lower quality or "incomplete" due to "missing" amino acids. However, the same 20 amino acids are used to build protein in plants as in animals and the genetic code is universal.[26-28] Vary your diet with veggies, seeds, nuts, grains and beans to get all the necessary macronutrients daily.

The DRI (dietary reference intake) for protein is about 0.36 grams per body weight pound (0.8 grams of protein per kilogram of body weight) for your body's basic needs and maintenance. For the average sedentary man, this equals 56 grams of protein per day and for the average sedentary woman, this equals 46 grams of protein per day.[27] This is sufficient to prevent a protein deficiency, but you can calculate your optimal protein intake based on activity level, muscle mass, age, current health and physique goals. There are a variety of free calculators and diets you can check out online, but I would recommend testing out a balanced plant-based diet, tweaking it over the next couple of weeks and see if you experience positive physical and mental changes. Continue reading for some general guidelines to get you started.

How much protein?

Protein is always of great concern for people when it comes to diet—perhaps the most commonly asked question, especially when it comes to a vegetarian or plant-based diet. So, how much protein should you be consuming each day? My suggestion is to aim for 0.36–0.6 grams of protein per pound of bodyweight and see how you feel.[26, 29] Please note, I would deviate towards the higher end if you are particularly active.

When I first started working out and tracking protein intake, I always ended up in a protein deficit, even before I started a plant-based diet. I was often confused because although I didn't *feel* bad physically, I couldn't wrap my head around the concept of "not getting enough protein" according to these calculators. I was constantly trying to figure out how much protein I needed in order to maintain or gain muscle mass, and the amounts seemed outrageous (often over 100 grams per day). At that time, I did find some information on when you should vary protein consumption, such as when you are trying to lose weight or gain muscle mass.

For weight loss, studies suggest 30% of your calories should come from protein to boost your metabolic rate and cause spontaneous reduction in calorie intake.[27, 30] A simple formula to calculate your protein intake if you're trying to lose weight is to multiply your calorie intake by 0.075. So, if you are eating a 2,000-calorie diet, that is approximately 150 grams of protein.

There are a lot of different suggested protein intake amounts when it comes to muscle gain and maintenance. Research largely recommends consuming 0.7–1 grams of protein per pound of lean muscle mass to gain mass. Keep in mind, lean muscle mass does not equal your weight.[27, 30]

You can figure out your lean muscle mass by searching "lean muscle mass calculator" on a search engine.

If you don't exercise much and are at a comfortable weight, aim for 0.36–0.6 grams of protein per pound. For the average male, that's about 56–91 grams of protein per day and for the average female, that's 46–75 grams of protein per day to maintain your weight.[27, 30]

Caloric intake

Personally, I'm not a fan of counting calories. I think it's stressful, toilsome and not fun. I'd rather try to eat as balanced of a diet as possible, get enough servings of the good stuff you need and call it a day. Nonetheless, if you like to track calorie consumption, as a general rule of thumb, males need 2,500 calories per day to maintain weight, and 2,000 calories per day to lose 1 pound per week, while females need 2,000 calories per day to maintain weight, and 1,500 calories per day to lose 1 pound per week.[27, 30]

Plant-based diet

Whether you're looking to lose weight, feel great or improve your overall well-being, I'd recommend switching to a whole food, plant-based diet. Whole foods come from minimally processed fruits, vegetables, grains and legumes. These natural superfoods can reduce and potentially eradicate most of your health problems and concerns.

Countless individuals are replacing their current diets with plant-based diets, from everyday people to professsional athletes. As I mentioned earlier, I first started learning about a plant-based diet when I was researching heart disease. Caldwell Esselstyn, M.D., a former Olympic rowing champion, compiled research on the benefits of adapting a low-fat, whole foods plant-based diet in his

2007 *Prevent and Reverse Heart Disease* book. This book is excellent and an easy read if you would like to delve deeper into the evidence behind the success of a plant-based diet to reduce and even reverse illnesses, including heart disease.[31]

Of course, at first, it might not seem so simple adopting a plant-based diet, especially when it comes to going to family, friends or business events that involve food (assuming there won't be very many vegetarian options). But, keep the end goal in mind and remember it's only as hard as you make it. You can always make it happen if you are truly invested in living your best life. After about 6–12 weeks, you will start experiencing positive changes, weight loss, improved well-being and your brain will downregulate the fat receptor over time, limiting your craving for fats. And once you start feeling better, you will want to stick to the diet. Don't knock it until you try it.

It's common sense when you think about it. Why would humans need milk from a cow, a completely different species? They don't. Why are humans the only mammal that continues to drink milk after they mature? Sort of counterintuitive in the grand scheme of things, don't you think? An ox is pretty powerful, right? Where does it get its protein? Plants. You need omega-3s from fish oil? Where do fish get omega-3s? Plants.

Yes, I know, any points I make can be countered with some beliefs you've learned over the course of your lifetime. Well, that's the beauty of science; you can support or refute anything if you procure the right evidence. However, with the evidence *I've* gathered, I would recommend a plant-based diet if you really care about your health, even if it's just temporary. You really have nothing to lose besides weight (if that's your goal) and misconceptions, but everything to gain!

More diet tips[32, 33]

- To juice or not to juice? I would recommend eating your food whole instead of juicing, as you lose the benefits of fiber when you juice fruits and veggies. Don't be lazy. It's not that much work to chew food. But if you're on a time constraint, juicing is better than no fruits and veggies at all.

- Fruit juice? Drinking fruit is like drinking straight sugar and can contain ingredients other than fruit. Eat it whole instead.

- If you start eating a plant-based diet and realize you're losing too much weight, eat more calories, larger portions, snacks, more protein-rich foods and whole grains. Listen to your body and stick to what works for you.

- Feeling tired and low on energy since switching diets? Make sure you're consuming enough calories! Eating more lentils, whole grains, starchy vegetables and beans will increase your caloric intake. Remember to work out because you need to use energy to make energy. Keep at it and you will start to feel better.

- Have some easy snacks such as almond packs or trail mix in your purse, car and backpack to avoid falling off of your diet in times of hunger. Plus, no one likes to be "hangry!"

- Carbs are not "bad." Your body burns through carbohydrates first, followed by protein, and lastly, fat. Understand the importance of balancing carbohydrates, proteins and fats to achieve your optimal health. It is more valuable to find a balance rather than to follow a yo-yo diet.

- I feel it's much better to buy seasonal over organic if you must choose one over the other due to price or availability. What you eat is more important than how it's produced. Therefore, if organic is too expensive, purchase conventional produce that's in season and move on with your life.

Plant-based foods[34-36]:

Nuts & Seeds:
- Almonds
- Cashews
- Chia seeds
- Coconuts
- Flaxseeds
- Macadamia nuts
- Peanuts
- Pine nuts
- Sunflower seeds
- Walnuts

Fruits:
- Apples
- Avocados
- Berries (strawberries, kiwifruit, blueberries, blackberries, raspberries)
- Citrus (oranges, grapefruit, mandarins)
- Pears
- Stone fruit (apricots, nectarines, peaches, plums)
- Tropical/exotic fruit (bananas, mangos)
- Melons (watermelons, cantaloupe, honeydew)

Vegetables:
- Asparagus
- Bell peppers
- Broccoli
- Brussels sprouts
- Butternut squash
- Cabbage

- Cauliflower
- Carrots
- Celery
- Corn
- Cucumbers
- Eggplant
- Garlic
- Kale
- Mushrooms
- Onions
- Peas
- Potatoes
- Spinach
- Sweet potatoes
- Tomatoes
- Zucchini

*By definition, some of these are fruits. However, fruits listed as veggies here are due to being closer to a vegetable when it comes to nutrition, cooking and USDA sites.

Whole Grains:

- Barley
- Brown rice
- Buckwheat
- Bulgar
- Freekeh
- Millet
- Oatmeal
- Popcorn
- Quinoa
- Sorghum
- Whole rye
- Wild rice

Beans:

- Black beans
- Cannellini beans
- Chickpeas
- Green beans
- Kidney beans
- Lentils
- Navy beans
- Pinto beans
- Soybeans

Dark Chocolate:

Dark chocolate is one of the most powerful sources of antioxidants and is full of magnesium. Enjoy in moderation with fruits and nuts if you'd like.

Use the pyramid below for creating quick meal plans and referencing daily serving sizes:

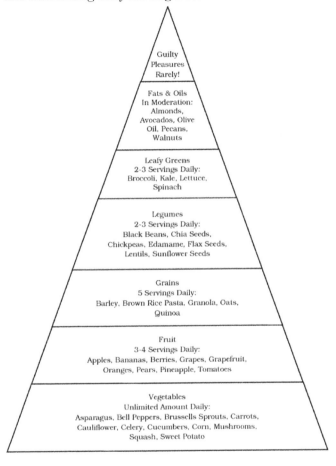

Dietary Reference Intakes

I know some people like to plan out exactly how much of everything they need. If you are one of these people, I recommend reviewing Dietary Reference Intakes (DRI), which refers to your body's nutrient requirements. The DRI—established by the Health and Medicine Division of the National Academies of Sciences, Engineering and

Medicine—calculates daily nutrient recommendations based on your height, weight, age and activity level.[27] You can use the calculator from the website below for individual estimates of Body Mass Index (BMI) and daily caloric needs, along with suggested intakes of macronutrients, vitamins and minerals.

DRI Calculator:
https://fnic.nal.usda.gov/fnic/dri-calculator/index.php

Water

We can all probably use more water. But how much do we *really* need? Well, it varies from person to person, climate conditions, different altitude levels, etc. Here's an idea: use common sense. Carry a refillable water bottle with you and sip on it throughout the day. When you're thirsty, drink water until you're not thirsty anymore. Drink more water when it's hot and when you exercise. Simple.

If you live in the U.S.A., adequate water intake is considered to be 2.7 liters (91 ounces) per day for women and 3.7 liters (125 ounces) per day for men. Please note, this is not just pure water, but water from all sources and includes water in your fruits, veggies, tea, etc.[37-41]Some signs that you should increase your water intake (or that you're dehydrated) include:

- Breath: dry and/or sticky mouth, bad breath.[41]
- Constipation: difficult or fewer bowel movements. Dehydration can cause and/or worsen constipation.[42]
- Thirst: self-explanatory.[38]
- Skin: chapped lips, less plump skin, rough or flakey skin.[41]

- Urine: dark yellow to amber color and ammonia smell; urine should be very light in color if you are sufficiently hydrated.[43]

Supplements

Many of us have dabbled in vitamins and supplements at some point. If you use the DRI calculator mentioned earlier, you may find you want to increase intake of a certain vitamin. Personally, I refrain from adding more stuff to worry about and try to keep things simple. I eat as balanced as I can, keeping it mostly plant-based, but do take vitamin B12 and vitamin D3. This is because I don't prefer most of the plant-based foods that are rich in vitamin B12 (tofu, nutritional yeast, soybeans, mushrooms) and don't spend a lot of time in the sun (to prevent premature aging).[44] Keep in mind, if you take supplements and are plant-based, they are not always completely vegetarian or vegan—many are encapsulated with gelatin. Gelatin is a protein, usually derived from swine or bovine bones, ligaments, tendons and skin boiled in water. It's also in most gummy bears, Jell-O and marshmallows. If this concerns you, be aware and always check ingredients.

If you decide to adopt a plant-based diet, it is crucial for you to take a vitamin B12 supplement because plants do not produce it. It is made by microbes that blanket the Earth, which are killed off in our water supply during the cleaning process. Vitamin B12 deficiencies can be extreme, with some cases resulting in paralysis, psychosis, blindness or even death.[45] These are some pretty serious reasons to supplement your plant-based diet with B12. It's an easy fix and you can take it once a week to get an adequate dose. If you are under 65 years old, you only need to take 2,500 mcg per week. As you age, absorption of vitamin B12 can decline, and it is recommended to up your dosage, perhaps up to 1,000 mcg of vitamin B12 daily. There are different forms of vitamin B12 and each has its advantages and disadvantages. I prefer to buy methylcobalamin because research shows it to be the most readily absorbed and stays in your system longer than other forms, while some people prefer the synthetic form of vitamin B12, cyanocobalamin. Both types can prevent vitamin B12 deficiencies.

If you are unable to get a sufficient amount of unprotected midday sun time each day, take a 2,000 IU vitamin D3 supplement with your largest meal.[45] I prefer taking a supplement over being in the sun during the peak hours, plus there are so many factors that go into getting the right amount of sun that depend upon the latitude, angle of sun rays, etc. It's just easier!

Summary

Nutrition is critical to your physical and mental health, which is why it is a huge part of this book. Make sure you eat a balanced diet, aiming to fill half your plate with fruits and vegetables every time you have a meal. Drink plenty of water, take the appropriate supplements and practice mindful eating.

Pillar II:
Social

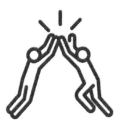

The Social Pillar of Wellness relates to building and maintaining meaningful relationships with others and knowing you are not alone. No matter what you've been through or what you've felt, there is someone out there feeling the same joy, pain, love, sorrow—whatever it might be—as you. This is simply a part of being human. Sharing experiences with others helps bond and build a sense of community, which generally leads to a more fulfilling, happier life. There are good people out there; you need to be aware of that so you can find more. Find people that share the same hobbies as you and expand your mind. Show the ones you love that you care about them often. Minimize your contact with those that bring you down.

Create healthy relationships wherever you can, with your family, friends, coworkers, community, as well as on social networks, if you use any. Surround yourself with people that bring you up, not down. If valuable relationships falter, try to repair them and learn to deal with conflicts appropriately. In the case you feel you do not have a strong network and want to meet new people, try to build new relationships by attending community events, volunteering or joining a recreational sports league. Always help others whenever you can, whether it's a random act of kindness or listening to a friend in need. Putting in the time and energy to create and maintain meaningful relationships is worth the effort and will serve you well in the long run.

Cultivate healthy relationships

Sure, making new friends isn't always easy; however, it is possible. If you find yourself looking for places to build new relationships, start with your interests. Do your hobbies include reading, sports, dogs or making a difference? Become a member of a book club, join a recreational sports team, go to the dog park or sign up to volunteer for a cause you believe in. Not feeling too peppy? Join a support group dedicated to an issue you're having— misery loves company. Just kidding. But really, if you have lost a loved one, have been through some major life changes or anything and you want to relate with other people, find a support group in your area. Sharing your experiences with others who have faced similar circumstances can be incredibly therapeutic and freeing. Learn to be friendly, open and nonjudgmental when you meet new people. Become genuinely interested—everyone has their own unique story. Take the time to practice active listening when others talk instead of focusing on what you have to say next or letting your mind wander. Having healthy relationships matters when it comes to living a long, happy and healthy life.

Nurture close relationships

It is easy to get caught up in today's fast-paced world, but nothing can replace the feelings of connecting with someone you care dearly about, whether it's a parent, a sibling or an old friend. Get into the habit of sending a text, leaving a voicemail, mailing a card or making a phone call to a few people each month to remind them you care and see how they're doing. There are plenty of ways to show others you care. It does not have to be a long, drawn out process or entail contacting 50 people at a time. Focus on a few people that matter most. Yes, this may take a little time, but a little time goes a long way when it comes to those that matter. In fact, research shows that having a healthy social network may help you live up to 50% longer.[1] Think quality over quantity when it comes to relationships—maintaining even three social ties can decrease your chance of early death by over 200%![2] On a physiological level, research shows healthy social circles are correlated with positive changes in the brain, the heart, hormones and immune function, reducing your risk of chronic illnesses.[3-7] Overall, nourishing valuable relationships can reduce your stress levels, improve immunity and extend your lifespan.

Learn to move on

There are countless variations of the saying, "Holding on to anger is like drinking poison and expecting the other person to die." In life, people will upset you. They may be strangers, significant others, coworkers, friends or family. Everyone copes with their anger differently, but it is important to pay attention to how much you invest into that anger. If you are angry with someone, learn to let the situation breathe, re-evaluate it and then come back to it with a cool mind. Practice positive problem-solving skills when it comes to conflict, and learn to forgive when necessary. In the end, anger and stress will only hurt you the most, so learn to keep your cool and not lose it over little things. If relationships falter, take the time to piece them back together when possible, if they truly matter. Keep in mind the only person you can change is yourself. You can only be responsible for your own actions. If someone upsets you and you cannot let go of things no matter how much time and discussion has passed, perhaps you should reevaluate the relationship.

Cut out the energy vampires

Perhaps you are feeling a little depleted or completely drained and you're not sure why. You're not hungry, got enough sleep, went for a nice little walk and your day started out great but something just feels exhausting and depressing. Do you start feeling this way around a particular person? Then you may be falling victim to an energy vampire—be it a best friend, family member, significant other, coworker or anyone else in your life. An energy vampire may be dominating, manipulative, narcissistic, constantly playing the victim and blaming others for problems, judgmental, a drama queen or someone who is legitimately helpless and used to leaning on others for support.[8]

Often times, energy vampires have deep rooted problems. You need to be aware of these types of people and understand that as much as you may want to help them, if they do not make any changes themselves and continue to harp on the same problems, it is an unproductive interaction, wasting time that could be spent otherwise, and will only bring you down. Here are some characteristics of an energy vampire:

- Has a low self-esteem, engages in self-pity, blames others for their problems, constantly has a "the world is out to get me" or "woe is me" mentality, without the humor
- Expects you to put them first, is self-centered, needs you to feed their ego and take orders, is manipulative, is dishonest, makes you feel disempowered, has a "my way or the highway" attitude
- Constantly creates problems to fill the emptiness in their life, loves drama because the negative emotions they feed off of become addictive, gossips and speaks poorly of others while making themselves look good
- Preys on others to buoy their own ego, attempts to make others feel small or bad about themselves, is judgmental, can be hypocritical
- Relies on you heavily for constant support, whether emotional or otherwise, because they are or feel helpless all the time

Instead of developing and having resentful feelings toward this energy vampire, learn to protect your peace and spirit. You may not be able to control others, but you are in control of how much time you spend with energy vampires or how you spend the time with them. There is no need to subject yourself to chronic anger, depression or anxiety. If the offender is someone you absolutely must be around, let them know you are trying to make positive changes in your life and would appreciate it if they helped by focusing on good things when you are around because it is difficult for you to improve yourself otherwise. The person may or may not understand—if you try and they ignore your wishes, you must find another way to deal with this situation. Limit your exposure to these types of people whenever possible, as much as possible. Do not take things an energy vampire does or says personally, for they are usually lacking self-awareness and self-worth. Treat them with kindness in the time you must be around them and refuse to participate in their negative behaviors, whether it is gossiping or pushing you around. If the person who drains you is naive and simply helpless, try to encourage them to be stronger and kindly remind them that you need time for yourself. Remember, you cannot help people that are unwilling to help themselves.

You will feel much better once you minimize your interactions with these people. It may not always be easy because you may have known some of these individuals for a very long time and feel strongly bonded to him or her. Trust me, I come from a place of experience when I say I know it isn't always easy to break free of certain people in your life, and I know it can take a long time. However, it is vital that you cut them loose if they affect you negatively. Disconnect and detox from them, even if it must be a temporary distance. Do not allow yourself to harbor negative feelings because of an energy vampire. You are on a new journey now. A journey to be the best version of you and need to surround yourself with those that inspire and uplift you, not the other way around. Be wise in choosing with whom you spend your time with. You are in control.

Pillar III:
Emotional

The Emotional Pillar of Wellness encompasses mood, confidence, demeanor, appreciating and cheering on others, showing gratitude, expressing emotions and realizing your full potential. You should be able to identify, analyze and share your feelings effectively. The way you carry yourself and communicate with others is imperative when it comes to feeling like a confident, stable person. People are not always good at reading others, expressing themselves or handling difficult situations appropriately. The good news is, there are many self-improvement tools, books and articles out there to assist in this department. Proper stress management can reduce emotions such as anger, frustration, anxiety and sadness when it comes to difficult situations. Read on for a few great guidelines.

Instant pick-me-up

Been feeling down in the dumps for a while and don't know how to get out? Try smiling, even if you're not in the mood for it. Your brain can be tricked into releasing dopamine with a fake smile, causing a boost in your mood, lower heart rate and decreased stress. Not in the mood to conjure up a smile? Then get physically active. It doesn't have to be a long gym routine; it can be as easy as jumping up and down or jogging in place. Your brain will begin to match your physical energy. Exercise is a natural depression fighter and will make you feel better. Be happy and spread the joy when you're happy. Laugh with others, at your mistakes and silly things. Life doesn't have to be that serious, so find the humor in it. Living a joyous life can boost your immune system, lengthen your life, combat pain and promote a generally healthier lifestyle.[1] You deserve to be happy, and by incorporating the 7 Pillars of Wellness into your life, you are taking a step in the right direction.

Be kind

Kindness has more power than you may know. It affects both you and others positively, with physical effects on your brain, heart, immune system and body. While stress releases stress hormones such as adrenalin and cortisol, kindness releases a "kindness hormone," known as oxytocin. Oxytocin makes you feel warm and connected to others, which is much different from stress hormones that work to lower your immunity. You can think of kindness as the opposite of stress because it has the opposite physical effects on your body compared to stress. For example, stress raises blood pressure while kindness reduces it; stress is detrimental to cardio-vascular health, while kindness protects your heart; stress can make people unhappy while kindness makes people happy; stress suppresses the immune system while kindness boosts it; stress tenses the nervous system while kindness relaxes it; stress increases inflammation while kindness reduces it; and stress can trigger depression while kindness can be an antidote for depression.

Moreover, research at the Yale School of Medicine has found stress to have an inverse relationship with kindness, meaning when kindness goes up, stress goes down. The more acts of kindness you do, the lower your stress levels and negative emotions will be. On the other hand, the less acts of kindness you do, the higher your stress levels and negative emotions will be.[2] Brain regions can grow when we exercise them, just like other muscles in our body. Therefore, if you focus on kindness over stress, the stress regions will shrink because you will not be using them as much—just like a muscle shrinks when you don't use it. The areas in your brain that focus on love, empathy and compassion will grow instead of the stress regions.

There is always more to someone than what meets the eye. Everyone has his or her own inner struggles and you may have no idea what someone is going through. Showing a small bit of compassion for someone else, whether or not you can relate, can make a huge difference in someone's life. Instead of looking down at your phone, look up at the people around you; a real human connection can never be replaced with a screen. Get into the habit of complimenting at least one person a day. You never know what a big difference something so small can make in someone's day, and it will make you feel good, too! Find something you genuinely like about someone and tell them—it can be someone's shirt, someone's energy or something else about them. Be careful when complimenting someone's appearance, especially in a business setting as it can often comes off as flirtatious. If someone lacks the ability to speak on their own behalf, be their voice. Making others feel good will give you a natural high and can have a ripple effect, spreading happiness and kindness. Be kind, because there is no reason not to be.

Use affirmations and positive self-talk

Boost your self-confidence, elevate your mood, improve your well-being and increase your overall satisfaction with yourself by using affirmations and positive self-talk. Find a good time to recite your affirmations and positive self-talk, whether aloud or in your head, in the morning, at bedtime or whenever you need them, and make it a habit. Little stickies can be used as reminders and placed on your mirror or door. Here are some wonderful affirmations to get you started[3]:

- Like the waves of an ocean, peace washes over me, cleansing and rejuvenating my spirit.
- I am grateful for my amazing life.
- I am confident and capable.
- All is always well.
- I feel so energetic and alive.
- I forgive and release. I am filling my heart and mind with love.
- I attract positive people in my life.

Positive affirmations and self-talk come in handy during times of need, such as when you feel overwhelmed or anxious. Use affirmations such as the ones above to write yourself a positive self-talk script. Studies have shown that positive self-talk can enhance the performance of athletes by aiding with endurance or powering through a set of heavy weights.[4] Positive self-talk can help you before a presentation or activity as well, since it is your inner dialogue. Your personality generally influences your self-talk, and if you are optimistic or pessimistic, it will influence your subconscious mind and expose your thoughts, beliefs, ideas and questions. If you have a negative outlook and inner dialogue, you can change it. Start by using the aforementioned affirmations to build your self-talk model. It's all about reframing. For example, instead of thinking, "I'm a failure and I embarrassed my-self," think "I'm proud of myself for trying and I'll do better next time. That took courage." Rather than thinking, "I'm out of shape and overweight. I'll never lose the extra pounds, so why bother," believe "I am strong and capable. I will get healthier because I want to and I can."

It is always possible to better yourself, but developing new good habits takes time and practice. To incorporate positive self-talk into your daily routine, recognize scenarios that trigger negative self-talk, such as being around a certain person or work events. This way you can anticipate a situation and can prepare beforehand. Once you are in the situation, take a minute to check in with yourself, and if you find yourself becoming negative, figure out how you can turn it around. Another way to help develop positive self-talk is to add more comedy to your life. Watch funny animal videos or your favorite comedian and surround yourself with positive people that make you smile. If your circle of friends is negative, you will absorb the pessimistic outlook and emotions of those around you, so reevaluate with whom you choose to spend your free time. Lastly, post stickies with positive words or affirmations around places you spend the most time in, such as your office or home. Some of us may be able to transform our negative self-talk to positive self-talk with minimal effort, while others may struggle a bit more and can seek help from a therapist to get back on the right track.

Learn to manage and release your emotions

Get into the habit of being happy for others, especially when they have something you may so badly want, such as a job promotion or relationship. Remind yourself what you may see on TV or social media isn't always what it appears to be. Someone so beautiful can have a dark emptiness looming inside of him or her, only to be concealed with an infectious smile. Avoid comparing yourself to others. Instead of being jealous of other people, be happy for them. Jealousy will never serve you and only affects you negatively. If someone has something you want or lack, let that inspire you. Realize the Universe is presenting you with images of what you want and aligns to attract anything you want, which includes negative energy. Choose to be inspired and celebrate what others have so the Universe will bring it to you too.

If you feel like you're on a roller coaster with life's ups and downs, learning to manage your feelings will make the ride a lot smoother. If discussing your problems with people in your life isn't working, talk to a therapist or a counselor. Or, if you prefer not to share your personal stuff with anyone at all, journal your thoughts and feelings. This way, you'll be able to quickly reference obstacles and successes during times of need. Furthermore, if you enjoy journaling, having a gratitude journal can be an amazing addition to your wellness journey toolkit. Each morning, write down at least one or two things you are grateful for. It can be anything. Being able to walk, having a bed, your toothbrush, your family, a job. Refer back to your gratitude journal whenever you need to remind yourself how blessed you really are and to attract more wonderful things into your life.

Be balanced

Remember, there are overlapping themes within the 7 Pillars of Wellness. They all work together to create the best version of you. For example, diet and exercise can help manage your negative emotions and bring new perspective on things. Instead of looking each pillar as an individual concept, look at each as they relate to one another. For the Social pillar, you will be happier if you create a strong social circle and practice compassion, volunteer and learn new things.

You will have good days and you will have bad days. Ups and downs are a part of our life experience. Even on your down days, go through the motions regardless of whether or not you're feeling great (unless you physically can't). Things will take time to change, but the important thing to remember is that it is all possible, and you *can* have it all. I believe in you!

PILLAR IV:
MENTAL

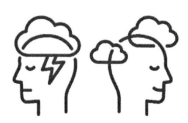

You are in control

One of the most significant things I'd recommend you remember is you are in control. You have the power to change your story by applying things you learn from this guide to become the best version of yourself. Nobody else can make that decision for you. You must learn the art of self-discipline and change your mindset.

Always grow

You may not always have time to sit down and read, but you can always listen to something in the background when you are working on tasks that don't require complete focus. You know what they say: "an idle mind is the devil's playground." I believe you should always be learning something because your brain is constantly hungry and will fall victim to boredom or begin to adopt undesirable characteristics if you starve it. If you don't have time to learn and grow, make time. For example, incorporate listening to a podcast during your morning routine while you are getting ready for the day. There is so much free motivation and education out there. Recently, I discovered the Mindset & Motivation podcast with Rob Dial— short, to-the-point podcasts that are usually about 15 minutes in length. Self-educate with audio books while you do dishes or clean at home. Listen to hypnosis instead of watching TV at night or when you're in bed. Everyone is always busy, but you can always make time for things that matter. You should matter.

Organized Surroundings = Organized Thoughts

Your surroundings affect your thought processes. If you are sitting amidst complete chaos, the disorganized environment can cause unnecessary stress and cloud your thinking. Physical and mental clutter get in the way of your flow, slowing down your ability to both move and think. Don't become a victim of the so-called "clutter effect" and clean up a bit—an untidy environment has a greater negative effect on you than you may realize.

For example, when you sit with piles of messy paperwork and everything is out of place, doesn't it feel overwhelming and uncomfortable? It makes it hard to know where to begin, right? Moreover, it's harder to find stuff, wasting time and creating frustration. Do yourself a favor and declutter your mind by cleaning up your home, office, backpack, purse, bag, car and living spaces. There's no need to stress and dig around to look for things all the time. If you're still not convinced, here are five reasons to make the changes, borrowed from Dr. Susan Krauss Whitbourne's article featured in *Psychology Today*[1]:

- **Improved subjective well-being**
  Living in clutter impedes how you identify with your

home. Your home should be a retreat from the outside world and a place to feel pride. A study conducted at the University of New Mexico found that having too many things in too small of a space will lead individuals to feel that their home environment is distressing, rather than a tranquil sanctuary.[2] Improve your subjective well-being by tidying up.

- **Healthier eating decisions**

An Australian-U.S. study conducted by Lenny Vartarian et al. (2017) showed that people will eat more cookies and snacks in a chaotic environment and end up feeling stressed. When researchers at Cornell University gave students cookies in a disorganized, messy, kitchen, students were put in a low self-control mindset and ate twice as many cookies as students in a standard, organized kitchen.[3] Make superior choices and regain control by decluttering your surroundings.

- **Better mental health**

University of South Carolina's Paul Bliese and colleagues discovered that in some of the first studies conducted on workplace stress, a comfortable environment was critical for "mental hygiene." Though recent research focuses more on mental comfort than physical comfort, conclusions from experiments on home cleanliness and organization can be applied to the workplace as well. Several experiments involving workplace satisfaction suggest that allowing employees to personalize their surroundings has a positive impact, but when surroundings become cluttered, diminishing returns result.[4] Boost your mental health by keeping your workspaces organized.

- **More efficient visual processing**

When your visual surroundings are cluttered with miscellaneous stimuli, it's more difficult to read what others are feeling. Cornell University's James Cutting and Kacie Armstrong conducted an experiment to discover how clutter affects perceptions on scenes in movies. Their work concluded viewers found it harder to interpret emotional expressions on faces of characters in highly cluttered movie scenes.[5] Should this apply to real life, it means you will have less accuracy when trying to analyze someone's true feelings if you are seeing them amidst a chaotic environment. Keep your visual processing performance at its best by keeping things organized.

- **Greater productive thinking**

"Mental clutter" can be defined as a "state of mind in which you can't inhibit irrelevant information." Lynn Hasher, a researcher at University of Toronto, has analyzed studies that support mental clutter as a prime suspect in causing age-related memory loss. The science behind this? If there is mental clutter blocking your neural networks, your information processing will be slower and less efficient. Consequently, your mind will lag when it comes to short-term memory tasks and even more in long-term memory exercises.[6] For instance, if you need to recall information you should know, such as names of people, you will be slower to find it "within your disorganized repository of knowledge" if your environment is unorganized. Let your thought processes flow smoothly by tidying up.

In conclusion, decluttering your spaces will have a positive impact on more than just your housekeeping. Decluttering plays a vital role in maintaining your happiness at home and work while simultaneously benefitting your physical health and cognition. Get rid of the extra stuff, whether it's tangible or virtual garbage, and feel the stress leave your body. Be at ease in your surroundings, think clearer and streamline your thought processes by keeping your spaces clean and organized.

Set goals, properly and practically

There are countless goal setting methods out there. One that is easy and to the point is known as "S.M.A.R.T." goals. Specific, Measurable, Achievable, Relevant and Time-bound. Writing out your goals is a great way to set up a road map for what to do next, keeps you on track and makes it more likely to be achieved. Get a pen and work through this exercise with me.

• Start out by writing out a general goal you would like to accomplish:

_____

_____

_____

_____

• Now get **S**pecific.

Relate your goal to something simple, sensible and significant. What do you desire to accomplish? Who needs to be involved? When and why do you want to do this?

Example: "I want to lose 10 pounds and tone up" is much better than "I want to get fit."

_____

_____

_____

_____

- Make sure the goal is **M**easurable.

  How will you measure your progress?

  Example: "I want to lose 10 pounds in the next 3 months."

  _____

  _____

  _____

  _____

- The goal should be **A**chievable and realistic.

  Do you need time to learn new skills before you can achieve the goal?

  Example: "I want to lose 10 pounds in the next 3 months and prepare for a marathon" is more realistic than "I want to lose 10 pounds and prepare for a marathon in 3 days."

  _____

  _____

  _____

  _____

- Have a **R**elevant, results-based goal.

  Make sure the goal aligns with your overall objective and achieving the goal will be worthwhile.

  Example: "Losing weight will help me prepare for a marathon and improve my overall health."

  _____

  _____

  _____

  _____

- Next, make the goal **T**ime-bound.
  Create a reasonable deadline.

  Example: "I will create a workout and diet plan within the next two days so I can lose 10 pounds in the next 3 months."

  _____

  _____

  _____

  _____

- Now, use the information you've written down and create a new S.M.A.R.T. goal statement.

  Example: "I want to lose 10 pounds in the next 3 months, prepare for a marathon and continue to improve my health over time because my body should be much better."

  _____

  _____

  _____

  _____

Visualize

I first discovered the power of visualization in a sports psychology course. It is a performance enhancing strategy that athletes use to improve skills by imagining detailed steps leading up to a victory. On a physiological level, as one envisions their perfect performance, the brain creates neural patterns as if the body were physically doing what is being imagined.[7, 8] What I really love is this technique is not limited to sports performance; you can apply this underutilized tool to various aspects of your life. Visualization is a powerful self-development tool because it adds emotion to your focus, boosting your motivation to achieve a goal. Whether your goal is to eat healthier, deliver a great toast or remain calm in a stressful situation, this technique can be applied.

Go into a situation with more confidence by doing a little homework beforehand. I won't delve too deeply into it, but here's a basic idea on how to visualize to enhance your performance:

- Find a quiet place. Maybe your bed, as you drift off to sleep.
- Take some deep breaths and get comfy.
- Close your eyes and think about the new behavior, skill, mood or goal.
- Imagine the situation or thing you want as clearly and as detailed as possible.
- Add emotion and sensation to your imagination.
- Visualize at least 10 minutes a day.
- Practice with a positive attitude and positive thoughts each time.

Try doing this with positive energy for a couple of days and feel your entire existence begin to change. The best part is, you don't need anything to do this besides your mind. Good luck with your hopes, dreams and aspirations... ask, believe and receive!

Don't multitask

I remember when putting multitasking under your skills was nearly equivalent to being proficient in Excel on resumes. Guess what? Multitasking causes brain drain and it's not all it's cracked up to be. It's most likely slowing you down, reducing your attention span and decreasing your productivity. I've analyzed several articles that explain how multitasking depletes cognitive resources and can lead to early mental decline, diminishing sharpness over time. Constantly switching between tasks increases your cortisol levels, possibly damaging the memory region of the brain. Allegedly, only 2% of people can successfully multitask. For the rest of us, it takes more time to switch from one task to another versus single tasking, so there's no point in wasting time trying to save time when you probably can't.

Chances are, you aren't going to increase efficiency and are more likely to make mistakes when you're multitasking anyway. Additionally, you might not even be multitasking by definition. Perhaps you're "serial tasking"—switching between multiple tasks quickly, like answering emails, taking calls and watching YouTube. How does that make anything faster? Numerous articles have cited a study that found you can lose 2.1 hours a day at work with office distractions![9-11] Do yourself a favor and don't overload your brain by inviting unnecessary stress into your life.

Relearning things and breaking old habits is a process, but not impossible. Let's make it simple by doing the following[12]:

- **Get rid of distractions**

Put your phone in an inconvenient location, mute unnecessary notifications, close extra windows and tabs on your computer, declutter your workspace and isolate yourself (as needed) to be productive. If possible, I would even turn the Wi-Fi off.

- **Set a deadline**

Part of what feeds the desire to multitask is lack of patience. Set some reasonably soon deadlines to finish what you need to do and see if that works. If it doesn't, then skip this step.

- **Focus**

Self-explanatory.

- **Take a break**

Get up, walk around, exercise, clear your mind, forget about what you're doing, and then come back to work on the task.

- **Repeat**

You might not be perfect the first time, especially if you're so used to trying to multitask. Stick to it and start experiencing significant stress reduction.

Take it one task at a time. Many of us create bad habits over time that eventually become second nature. By using the multitasking detox strategy from above, you can recondition your brain to overcome multitasking syndrome and actually be more productive.

Hypnotherapy

Hypnosis can be an excellent, effective self-improvement tool. Most people are only aware of the type of hypnosis used for entertainment. However, there is a clinical type of hypnosis that can be used for medical purposes. Strong evidence supports hypnosis being successfully used for the treatment of pain, irritable bowel syndrome, post-traumatic stress disorder and insomnia. The efficacy of hypnosis to treat depression, anxiety, smoking cessation, post-surgical wound healing and weight loss varies from case to case, with limited research and evidence, but is worth a try.[13-15] Researchers have found that distinct regions of the brain that play roles in action control and awareness are altered while undergoing hypnotherapy.

These studies suggest the brain reacts to hypnosis in a way stronger than a placebo effect.[16]

Hypnotherapy is the practice of using hypnosis for therapeutic purposes. Here's how it works: during hypnosis, verbal cues and repetition will guide you into a trance state—a state of deep relaxation, hyper focus, concentration and increased suggestibility. Once in trance state, you may experience sleepy symptoms but will be fully aware of what's happening. At this time, the trained hypnotist or hypnotherapist will make guided suggestions to help you reach your goals. Your mind will be in a heightened state of focus, potentially making you more open-minded to advice or proposals that you may otherwise disregard in your normal state. The session will end either when you wake from the trance state on your own or by the therapist waking you from it. A single session may be helpful for one person, whereas someone else might need more or some maintenance sessions for the hypnosis to be effective.[17] I encourage anyone that may be interested or curious to check out some guided hypnosis podcasts available online or through apps on your phone.

I believe hypnosis can be a powerful tool to make positive changes in your life. In the past, I have listened to the Joseph Clough Hypnosis app, which is filled with tons of free content that is very useful. Joseph Clough's pod-casts are focused on changing your mindset to overcome obstacles in your life. Sure, everyone can't be hypnotized (and likely not by using an app or over the internet), but this is still a great app to use as a motivational podcast or to train up your mind. The whole point of trying different things with the same goal in mind is to discover strategies that work effectively for you.

Invest in your health

Don't waste your money on silly stuff. You might not realize how much extra spending you're doing until it's brought to your attention. This can relate to items you don't really care for and impulsively buy, adding to your pile of clutter. Or, it can be spending the $5 every day on a coffee when you could save both time and money by making your own. If you make your own, you have more money to spend on healthy stuff. Plus, you can get a higher quality product that you hand pick. When buying things that aren't necessities, decide whether or not it will really bring you joy and for how long. Ask yourself if you need it and question the quality of it before you buy it. If it's something of low quality that you will have to replace soon, perhaps you should opt to wait, save up and get a higher quality product that will last longer. There's no reason to be wasteful with your finances and stress over them later. Something to think about.

You can make all the excuses in the world to not make life changes, one often being not having money for a gym membership or healthy foods. It is still possible to get healthy and fit. The key is finding ways to do it. For instance, you don't need a gym membership to work out. There are countless home bodyweight workouts you can do at home and outdoors. If you feel you don't have enough money for healthy food, you can reevaluate your spending habits and try to move some money around. You may be purchasing a coffee every morning for $5 when you could buy a box of 50 organic green tea packets or something similar for the same price, which will not only save you time and money, but also last a long time. Think about it—if you spend $5 every day on a drink, that's $35 a week, $140 a month, $1,680 a year on a coffee. You can put that $35 a week towards your grocery budget. There are several YouTube videos on how to eat well on a budget; all you need is to run a quick search. We live in a time where there is so much free information at the tip of your fingers—use it to your advantage! See where you can cut down expenses. You might be spending on monthly subscriptions you don't even use that are set on auto-renew. Sell things you don't need or use. Down-sizing can be a very freeing, uplifting feeling. Invest in your health now so you don't have to pay for it later. I repeat, invest in your health now so you don't have to pay for it later!

Minimize stress

Most of us experience stress from time to time, some more than others. One must know how to manage it and retrain the mind so that it doesn't affect the body negatively. I like to channel negative feelings of stress, sadness and anger through working out, listening to music or a favorite podcast, going for a long walk, spending time with my dog or writing poetry. A lot of people like to meditate or practice yoga to quiet their mind, which are also great options. The possibilities are endless on how you can redirect that negative, stressful energy into something positive that you enjoy. Yell at the top of your lungs if it makes you feel better. (Don't strain your vocal cords too much!) Sometimes, you just have to let it out and reset. Consider what makes you feel good and learn to put your mind at ease.

Keep your goal in mind

Always keep your end goal in mind. Focus on what can go right instead of what can go wrong. The more you focus on something, the more of that thing your subconscious mind will bring you. For instance, when you desire a certain car, you start seeing it everywhere. When you learn a new word, you start hearing it more. It's not that these things didn't exist before, they just weren't on your radar. Think of it this way: when you are trying to get somewhere unfamiliar, you enter the desired destination into your GPS and that's it. You don't put in all the places you don't want to go, because they don't matter. Rather than focusing on everything that can go wrong on your way to reaching your dreams, focus only on where you're headed. Keep your eye on the prize.

Stay motivated

You have to make a decision for yourself, because no one else is going to push you the way you need to be pushed. Do you really want this? Are you ready to make yourself a priority? Sure, you might say you don't have time to go to the gym, do grocery shopping, whatever, but how about all the people who say that and end up getting sick? Somehow, they make time and pay thousands of dollars to go to the doctor's office when they *need* to. You *need* to make changes now, so you don't end up that way. If you are already dealing with health problems, whether mental or physical, then it's time to learn to manage your life better. Stop making excuses. It's your responsibility to continue to motivate yourself, so read inspiring books, listen to podcasts, work out hard, write yourself notes, do whatever it takes! Find someone or some way to keep yourself accountable.

Be realistic

It's not the end of the world if you slip once and have a cookie after a week of healthy eating. You have to reward yourself while you change your habits. When people take on extreme diets or routines, they generally tend to fail because it's not practical and may feel depriving. It's demotivating when you feel like you're failing. If you miss one or two days at the gym, don't stop going indefinitely. There is no need to concentrate on what happened when you can make something better happen now, by getting back in there as soon as possible. Find a balance; don't obsess over the little things and live your life. The journey of health and fitness is always fluctuating. It's all about balance. It's not the end of the world if you mess up once.

Practice self-discipline. Think of the end goal. Condition your mind to imagine how you want to be, look and feel until you get there. Act as if you are already that way. If you're walking down an aisle of temptation, remind yourself of your end goal. You're not weak, you can do this. Sweets will tempt you, but the satisfaction won't be so sweet, it'll be short-lived! Always keep the end goal in mind and visualize that whenever you feel tempted. For example, if your skin breaks out when you eat sugary or fried food, remind yourself of the negative side effects if need be, and focus heavily on how you will have fresh, clear skin after choosing a healthier alternative. Imagine being that beautiful, confident version of yourself. Act like who you want to become, right now.

Choose your words wisely

Words matter. In psychology, there is a concept known as priming in which you unconsciously react to words or images in positive or negative ways. For example, in the book *Blink*, Malcom Gladwell describes a study where researchers asked subjects to take a sentence completion test, subtly slipping in words such as old, Florida, wrinkled, wise, Bingo. The result? Participants left the experiment walking at a slower pace, feeling a bit more tired. Unbeknownst to them, their subconscious minds picked up clues in the conversation that made it appear that they were in an environment really concerned about aging, so they acted accordingly.[18]

Your subconscious mind is always eavesdropping on your deepest thoughts. In seconds, your unconscious mind can pick up small details without you realizing it so that you can focus on the matter at hand, which is exactly why the words you speak and give in to are so important. So, if you focus on words such as terrible, horrible, mad and angry, you will attract more negative feelings and things into your life; whereas if you focus on words such as laughing, joy, good health, love, happiness and excitement, you will attract more positive things into your life. The words you hear, taste and inhale will prime you and affect the way you behave. Choose them wisely.

Write your own story, create your own world

Every day, we are bombarded with ridiculous media images that are truly deceptive. The world is not full of hate, people don't have perfectly airbrushed bodies in real life and you don't have to give in to the belief that members of the opposite sex are all terrible. There is no need to absorb this stream of trash. Try to feel genuinely good about yourself and be secure in who you are. Don't waste your life reading someone else's script, write your own. You are the movie star of your own life and have the power to create, direct, write and rewrite your story however you choose. Create a world you love and want to live in. Shut out the rest. For example, if you believe that people are generally bad because you are exposing yourself to this concept through the media, discussing it with others and starting to believe it, you will attract more bad people into your life. Everyone is not the same. There are good people in the world, and in order to attract them, you need to focus on them. If you see everyone in a negative light, that is what your subconscious mind will find you more of. It's all about the Law of Attraction—a basic principle that you attract anything your mind focuses on. *The Power*, by Rhonda Byrne is an excellent read if you want to learn more about the Law of Attraction or just want to get into a positive mindset.

Summary

The Mental Pillar of Wellness is essentially self-awareness, conditioning your brain, increasing intelligence and properly managing stress. Keep your mind sharp by reading, playing brain games and always strive to inspire and challenge yourself. Sign up for some classes you find interesting at your local community college or university, visit your local library, watch videos on topics with which you are unfamiliar, get involved in community activities. Take care of your mental health and stay motivated.

Pillar V:
Spiritual

The Spiritual Pillar of Wellness relates to your overall purpose in life and is based on your inner peace, values, beliefs and faith. Spend time to worship (whomever or whatever you believe in), reflect and meditate. Go out and connect with nature, breathe in some fresh air and take in the vivid colors, sights and sounds of the wonderful world we live in. Having purpose helps maintain perspective and overcome challenges. We each have our own purpose and that includes attracting whatever we want in life. In other words, keep your inner spirit alive and well.

Spiritual practices such as meditation, yoga, deep breathing, relaxation, reflection and prayer are excellent stress management techniques that help you see things from a different perspective. It is important to feed your spirit in order to grow as a person, become resilient in times of adversity and heal from past or present hurts, whether physical or mental. There is no "right" way to practice spirituality, as it serves the same purpose— calming and centering yourself. Some may express their spirituality through serving their community while others may seek solace in quiet ponderings in nature. Perhaps you would like to do both. Create your own ritual to reflect and reset by taking time out at least 10 minutes a day to re-center yourself. There are no rules when it comes to building your best life.

Meditate

Does your typical morning start with some sort of variation of this scenario: hit the snooze button followed by setting yourself on autopilot as you proceed to drink some coffee, scroll through your phone while eating breakfast and head out for the day? If so, instead of such an undesirable way to coast through your morning in a frazzled-zombie mode, try to start each day with some meditation. You can meditate while you make your bed each morning. It can be part of your morning ritual to wake up your senses. Fluff your pillows and fold the blankets. Sit quietly for a moment. It shouldn't take more than five minutes of your 24-hour day. Such a small task can encourage you to conquer larger tasks. Make it relaxing and set the tone for the rest of your day.

Meditation is great for stress reduction, anxiety management, relaxation and improving symptoms for stress-related illnesses such as post-traumatic stress disorder and irritable bowel syndrome. Furthermore, meditation improves mindfulness, patience, and self-awareness.[1] Large-scale studies conducted on thousands of people suggest meditation reduces the inflammatory response to stress, which can include restless sleep, higher blood pressure, depression symptoms, anxiety symptoms and clouded thinking.[2,3] You can practice the art of meditation anywhere, without any equipment, which is all the more reason to try it out.

There are different types of meditation. Two types you

may want to consider are focused-attention meditation and open-monitoring meditation. Focused-attention meditation brings your attention to a single object, thought, sound or visualization to encourage ridding your mind of distractions. Some focal points can be breathing, a mantra or a soothing sound. Open-monitoring meditation emphasizes increased awareness of all attributes of your sense of self, thought process and environment.[4] Perhaps you will find you like both types and decide to switch off. This is fine because there are no rules when it comes to how you meditate.

I would recommend incorporating meditation into your daily routine by waking up a few minutes earlier than usual in the morning to find some quiet time before, during or after you make your bed. This can encourage you to get into the habit of starting your day calmly. If you prefer to start with some guidance, there are free guided meditations available online on various websites, including the UCLA Health website where you can play an audio or read a transcript for meditations in as short as five minutes. If you choose to be on your smartphone early in the morning, there are apps like Headspace and Insight Timer you can use for your meditation sessions. Look into it to see what you like. Alternatively, if you find it difficult to get some quiet time and space to yourself, consider signing up for a class. The supportive environment will help with your meditation goals and get you started.

Spend time in nature

Boost your mental and physical health by spending at least 120 minutes a week in nature. A recent study surveying over 19,000 individuals in the United Kingdom revealed better self-reported health and wellbeing in those that spent time in nature compared to those that did not spend any time in nature. Regardless of whether individuals spent the 120 minutes taking short walks, hanging out at the park or going on long hikes, everyone benefitted from spending time outdoors.[5] Additional studies have found short periods of time in nature can provide great health benefits as well, even if it's only exercising for just five minutes outside—great for boosting your self-esteem and mood.[6] It's very easy to do, just step outside for a second. Once you are outdoors, make sure you give nature your undivided attention. Put down your smartphone or you will not reap the full benefits of nature's prescription. Try to take breaks outside whenever you can, if the weather permits. It's a great time to stretch and relax a little. After all, that's what breaks are for, to let you recharge!

One of my favorite ways to get in touch with my spiritual side is to go for a nice hike. It's refreshing to breathe in the scent of fresh trees, be rejuvenated by the sun and find a quiet place to relax and reflect. I love to take in all the vibrant colors, sounds and smells (hopefully good!) when I am outdoors and appreciate the often forgotten exquisite beauty that surrounds us. I try to feel the presence of the plants, animals, streams and sky around me. If there is a space I am drawn to, I will stretch and stand there for a few minutes as I embrace being amongst the trees, hills and mountains. The physical activity involved in hiking is just an added benefit of being out in nature. Always make sure you pack water and a snack if you plan on being out long. Although you can be more introspective when you are in nature by yourself, there is nothing wrong with sharing the experience with someone else, especially if you are not comfortable wandering into nature alone. Just make sure you set aside time to meditate on your own at some point!

Take your time

Learn to slow down. We don't realize how quickly time goes by until it has already gone. Rather than going through the motions day in, day out, learn to enjoy the little things. Here is a poem I came across, long ago, that may bring things into light for you...

Slow Dance by David L. Weatherford[7]

Have you ever watched kids on a merry-go-round,
or listened to rain slapping the ground?

Ever followed a butterfly's erratic flight,
or gazed at the sun fading into the night?

You better slow down, don't dance so fast,
time is short, the music won't last.

Do you run through each day on the fly,
when you ask "How are you?", do you hear the reply?

When the day is done, do you lie in your bed,
with the next hundred chores running through your head?

You better slow down, don't dance so fast,
time is short, the music won't last.

Ever told your child, we'll do it tomorrow,
and in your haste, not see his sorrow?

Ever lost touch, let a friendship die,
'cause you never had time to call and say hi?

You better slow down, don't dance so fast,
time is short, the music won't last.

When you run so fast to get somewhere,
you miss half the fun of getting there.

When you worry and hurry through your day,
it's like an unopened gift thrown away.

Life isn't a race, so take it slower,
hear the music before your song is over.

Pillar VI: Physical

In addition to proper nutrition, you should pay special attention to your physical body; this means you must maintain proper hygiene, get adequate rest and exercise daily. Try a variety of different types of exercises to figure out what you like best. It can be intimidating to start working out after a long time, or even for the first time ever. But it's really not that hard! All you need are some comfy clothes, water and space. Here is a short list of ideas on how to get active:

- Walking
- Gardening
- Swimming
- Yoga
- Aerobics
- Skating
- Jumping jacks
- Housework
- Biking
- Playing sports
- Hiking
- Weightlifting
- Dancing
- Running
- Jump roping
- Bodyweight exercises
- Skiing
- Rock climbing
- Jogging
- Pull-ups/push-ups

Put your phone away

Some of us are motivated while working out when we have an incredible soundtrack playing in the background. While there's nothing wrong with this, I often notice people taking up space at the gym, wasting time sitting on benches scrolling through their phone. If you want to do that, do it in a different area. If you use your phone while working out to listen to music or audio, that's completely fine, as long as you're not checking it every time you complete a set or focusing on your phone more than your body movement. Don't let it become a counterproductive habit.

I have started leaving my phone in a locker when I work out at the gym. I'll listen to one song that I'm really feeling to get me amped up before I walk in. When I'm working out, I want to focus on working out. Since I adopted this habit, I've reduced time spent in the gym and realized I was wasting precious time doing useless stuff on my phone. Think of it this way: athletes don't whip out their phones every five minutes to check messages, dating apps, social media or to change the music when they're in the middle of a game. They are concentrating on the task at hand. Try to exercise with that mindset. Stop wasting time and focus on that mind-body connection to make your workouts more effective.

Wipe down machines and wash your hands

Let's be real. If you're working out at a gym, it's a public place and it's not going to be a sterile environment. In fact, a study by a company called FitRated found an exercise bike to have 39 times more bacteria than a plastic reusable cafeteria tray, a treadmill to have 74 times more bacteria than a water faucet and free weights to have 362 times more bacteria than a toilet seat![1] That being said, make sure you wipe down machines before and after use or at the very least, avoid touching your face during your workout and wash your hands thoroughly at the end of your workout. To minimize contact with machines and weights (especially during flu season), try to wear work-out gloves, which also help with grip, and lay down a towel whenever you sit or lie on a bench, yoga mat or machine. Make sure you wash the gloves and towel regularly.

Comparison can be the thief of joy

It can be natural to scan the gym as you walk in. Perhaps you notice there are a lot of fit people already working out. For some, this can cause anxiety and comparison thinking: "I can never look like that," "he or she is already so fit and doesn't even need to work out," "what am I even doing here?" Stop right there! So what? If anything, being surrounded by fit people should inspire you to be a stronger, fitter, more confident version of yourself. Everyone has their own issues, probably including the person you are comparing yourself to, so stop worrying about other people and focus on yourself. You are there for a reason and that is to improve your health, not to subject yourself to emotional bullying. Get rid of that high school mentality and get to work. Put in the effort and you too shall succeed.

Find out how you exercise best

Many people gravitate towards group fitness over solo gym workouts because it builds a sense of community, provides expert guidance from an instructor, spices things up and makes the workout fun. Working out with others or having a workout partner increases accountability and motivation. It's all about trying out different things and finding what works for you—whether it's starting out your fitness regimen with a light walk after a meal, going for a hike with your dog, attending a group fitness dance class or hitting the gym solo. Take the time to try out a variety of activities to see which one makes you happy. Or mix it up every few months to keep things fresh and interesting. Decide when the best time for you to exercise is. Is it the morning when you have a lot of energy, the afternoon to get that second wind or the evening to wind down? There are no rules when it comes to how and when you have to work out.

What to put in a gym bag?

It's always useful to have a gym bag ready to go, especially if you're squeezing in a workout during a lunch break or right after work. Here are some handy things you can equip your gym bag with:

- Water bottle
- Weightlifting gloves
- Towel
- Deodorant
- Lock for locker
- Extra socks
- Gym shoes
- Workout clothes
- Hair ties
- Jump rope
- Snack, like a protein bar or trail mix

Pre and post exercise nutrition

Here's a little overview of eating habits in relation to your exercise schedule. For optimal performance, you should eat a full meal two to three hours prior to your workout. If you're eating closer to your workout, opt for a smaller snack with some simpler carbs and protein.[2] In regards to post-workout nutrition, eat a meal within 45 minutes of your workout.[3] It is important to eat prior to your workout to maximize your performance and minimize muscle damage, and equally important to eat post workout to replenish depleted energy stores and rebuild muscle.[4, 5] You can maximize your performance and improve your body composition by using these guidelines.

Don't sit too long

In this day and age, having a desk job is nearly the gold standard when it comes to work life. However, did you know over forty studies have discovered that excessive sitting causes irreversible damage to your body, decreasing your lifespan regardless of whether or not you exercise for an hour a day? The American Cancer Society conducted a fourteen-year study on over 100,000 men and women, finding men that sat more than six hours a day had a 20% higher chance of death compared to those that sat less than three hours a day, and women that sat more than six hours a day had a 40% higher chance of death compared to those that sat less than three hours a day.[6]

If your job requires you to sit all day, fret not, all hope is not lost, for life always has options. If you have the luxury to use a treadmill or standing desk, do so. Suggest having walking meetings, whenever possible. Studies have proven that interruptions that get you off your booty throughout the day are beneficial, even if it's just standing up at your desk for a minute at a time. There are plenty of desk exercises you can perform throughout the day such as chair dips and seated leg lifts.

Foam roll

Foam rolling is an exceptional form of self-massage and can be used for:[7]

- Alleviating soreness
- Improving mobility and overall wellbeing by increasing blood flow and elasticity in connective tissue (muscle tissue, joints, fascia)
- Helping prevent injuries by loosening tension and tightness in muscles while maintaining their length
- Reducing inflammation post workout
- Aiding in muscle repair recovery

It's a good idea to foam roll before a workout to warm up or exercising to prevent soreness. Those who sit for prolonged periods of time, have poor posture, improper form while working out or joint issues can also benefit from foam rolling. Foam rollers can cost under $10 and are a great investment to add to your exercise toolkit. An added perk is foam rollers are excellent for relaxation! Keep one around wherever you spend a lot of time so you can roll your way into relaxation.

Massages

Whether you prefer deep tissue massages, self-myofascial release or a soothing spa massage, they all have fantastic physical and psychological advantages when it comes to relaxing and treating muscle pain. Massages can aid in reducing muscle tension and inflammation, increasing blood flow and improving flexibility, particularly between workouts. You don't need to go to a fancy spa to reap the benefits of massage. You can use a foam roller, TheraCane or other self-myofascial release tools at home. These are inexpensive instruments that can be used at your convenience and provide amazing relief. There are several techniques you can use to target specific issues, such as neck tension or low back pain, which you can quickly look up online. Discover your favorite massage style by trying some out.

Summary

The Physical Pillar of Wellness focuses on your physical body. Focus on eating healthy, good hygiene, exercising and getting enough sleep. Brush and floss daily. Keep your body clean and fresh. Make time to go for a walk if you are too busy to do a proper workout that day. Maximize your quality of sleep by avoiding screens 30 minutes before bedtime, create a nightly wind down routine (dim lights, play calming music, shower, stretch) and block out unnecessary light before you get in bed.

PILLAR VII:
INTEGRITY.

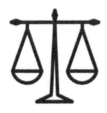

Carry yourself with integrity. Integrity is when you are the best version of yourself by being genuine and adhering to strong values. Your set of morals and values do not have to originate from religious practices, although they may if that is what you prefer. Learn to be self-aware of your physical body. For example, you may not realize while you were fully consumed by your cell phone that you nearly bumped someone walking your way. Chew with your mouth closed. Keep your promises and practice exceptional manners. There are plenty of ways you can enrich your life by working on your personal integrity.

When it comes to having integrity, one must always be honest, loyal and authentic. Do the right thing when no one is looking, without expecting acknowledgement. Treat others with kindness and hold yourself accountable. There is no reason to judge someone who does not have the same beliefs as you. We are all different and you cannot control anyone besides yourself, nor should you try to. Return things you borrow. Don't keep secrets from your spouse or partner and always remain true. Practice empathy and be compassionate towards others. Try doing random acts of kindness. You don't have to do something extravagant to brighten someone's day; it can be as simple as holding the door open for the person behind you. Always try to uplift those around you. When someone tells you something in confidence, respect their privacy and do not gossip.

Polish your verbal and non-verbal communication skills, be comfortable saying no in situations that you feel necessary, learn proper etiquette and avoid those who lack integrity, whether in business or personal life. Be a human of great integrity, as it is a very respectable trait to have. Some say integrity is hard to define, but you know it when you see it. Do you agree?

Superb manners never go out of style

Always practice proper etiquette. Simple phrases such as "thank you," "may I please…" "excuse me," and "I'm sorry" can go a long way and should never be forgotten. Having good manners has many advantages, including setting a good example for others (especially for your children), receiving positive attention in professional environments, maintaining romantic and nonromantic relationships due to mutual respect, and earning reciprocated kindness and respect. In addition, it can increase your confidence in situations because you won't be worrying about saying or doing the wrong things. Great manners will make a good impression because it shows others you are considerate and respectful of their feelings.

During conversation, maintain eye contact, avoid using profanity, practice active listening and don't interrupt the other person. At the table, place your napkin in your lap, wait until everyone is served before starting to eat, chew with your mouth closed and keep anything non-food related off the table—this includes your phone. If you must use your phone, excuse yourself and go to the restroom to check it. Be self-aware when you are out and about; if you accidentally bump someone, apologize and move on. Don't drag your feet slowly when others are tailgating you on the sidewalk. Move so they can pass. If you arrive at a door before the other person, you should open it. Send thank you notes or messages to show your appreciation if someone does something nice for you and congratulate others on their accomplishments. If you make eye contact with a stranger, don't stare too long because it can come off as creepy, weird, rude and uncomfortable—especially when males do this to females. When you run into someone you know and are with someone who does not know the other person, introduce them to each other before carrying on a conversation (and don't keep the person you are with waiting too long). Even if those around you don't practice good manners, you should. Stop spending time with those who consistently lack good manners.

Be humble

Arrogance is a characteristic that never shines in a positive light. Regardless of how successful, attractive, rich or better you feel than another person, there is no need to showcase it. While there is nothing wrong with being proud, it serves you better to remain humble. Realize that not everyone has had the same advantages as you, and bragging will only reflect poorly upon yourself. Likewise, there is no need to spend money to be flashy and impress others because that doesn't show your true merit. Don't judge others if they have different back-grounds, religious beliefs or economic status than yours.

If you run into an acquaintance or someone you know, say hello even if you are in a rush—you merely need to acknowledge their presence and can move on quickly. Those who choose to gossip paint a poor reflection of themselves—avoid it. Never ask someone personal questions such as how much they pay for things or about their domestic affairs. Mind your own business. In a nutshell, "Do unto others as you would have others do unto you."

Your word is your bond

"My word is my bond," denotes one will do what one has promised to do. It is important to follow through on commitments. There's no reason to make promises you cannot or do not plan to keep—why build the reputation of being flakey and unreliable? To avoid this shortcoming, when someone asks you to do something, before jumping to a yes or no, pause and think about it, whether you can, want to, and will follow through. Sure, there will be times when you are sick or something comes up and you cannot follow through with a commitment. There is no shame in that. Learn to cancel with grace; admit you've over-committed, let the other party know you are sick or something serious has come up, whatever it might be, in a timely manner, whenever possible. As long as this isn't a regular occurrence, it shouldn't be an issue. If you are known to make empty promises or not come through when you claim you will, then it is time to make a change.

Don't be a constant complainer

Sure, things don't always go the way you want them to and you might complain. While there is nothing wrong with complaining once in a while, it becomes an unattractive trait when you are constantly complaining. If you need to vent about something, allow yourself no more than five minutes. Get it out and move on. Don't continue to bother multiple people about how your coffee came in late this morning and you lost a sock—no one cares, seriously. It's annoying and negative if you keep doing it. There is no need to give so much attention to trivial things in your life, things that are out of your control or minor inconveniences. Remove chronic complainers from your life, become aware of your own complaining, catch yourself as you start to do it and learn to stop and redirect your thoughts. The more you complain, the more negative energy you are going to create and attract. No one wants to be around that.

Learn to be diplomatic

Another aspect of having great integrity is being able to maneuver sticky situations by being diplomatic. There is no need to argue over disagreements. Everyone will have their own opinion and there will be people who believe they know everything about everything and are never wrong. When one is diplomatic, they are able to evaluate a situation before speaking or reacting in order to take the best course of action while remaining composed and tactful. Always aim for win-win solutions.

When you approach the situation, make sure you choose you words carefully, especially in sensitive situations. Use "I feel…" or "I think…" type statements over accusatory statements that start with "you," as they usually put the other party in a defensive position. View things from the other person's perspective to try to get an insight on how he or she feels and what the best solution for both parties is. Be open to new ideas and do not be aggressive or overly authoritative; instead, use indirect language and encouragement to get something done. Make sure you start with a positive comment before delivering bad news, mind your manners, control your emotions and never yell. These are just a few ways you can be diplomatic in stressful situations, but you can always research more on your own.

Improve your social skills

Part of having high integrity is possessing the ability to communicate your message effectively through verbal and nonverbal communication when you connect with people. If you are not a social person by nature, the good news is you can learn to be one. Practice by starting small and simply acting social. Try to spark up a casual conversation with people you encounter, such as someone standing next to you in line, or just say "hi" to someone walking by. Ask open-ended questions that cannot be answered with a simple yes or no, such as "How do you feel about…?" Give genuine compliments and get people to talk about themselves. Practice being interested in what others have to say—everyone has their own unique story and you may find something in common to discuss afterwards. Pay attention to your body language as well; use the right amount of eye contact, avoid fidgeting, face the person during conversation and appear open to conversation, of course. Not sure what to talk about? Stay up to date with current events, but avoid controversial topics. Start to gather knowledge on an array of topics so you can find something to talk about with most people. Or, ask about places the person has lived before, where he or she grew up, what he or she liked to do growing up, etc. This is just a start, but there are several books on how to improve your social skills, and blogs you can look up with tips and tricks to get started.

"Without integrity and honor, having everything means nothing."—Robin Sharma

Always do the right thing, even when no one is watching, and expect nothing in return. Trustworthiness is the only way to gain honor and without it, you have nothing. When you have a reputation of being trust-worthy, your words and actions are of extraordinary value because you never waste time making excuses for not following through or forgetting your promises when other situations make it convenient to do so.[1] Endeavor not to choose temporary pleasure over what will result in broken trust, disloyalty, or hurt someone you love. If you feel you do not want to be with someone any longer or it's just not working, it is better to let him or her go first rather than making matters more complicated.

What are your thoughts on the 7 Pillars of Wellness?

Dear Reader,

First and foremost, thank you for purchasing *The 7 Pillars of Wellness*. I know self-help, wellness and health books are far and plenty, but you chose this book, for which I am very grateful.

I really hope this book has benefitted and improved your everyday life. If so, please take some time to review it on Amazon. I value your feedback and support. Feel free to spread the love and share this book through social networks, such as Facebook, Instagram and Twitter. Wishing you all the best in your health and happiness goals!

Sincerely Yours,
 -Sasha

YouTube: www.youtube.com/MissSashaDeol
Twitter: @MissSashaDeol
Instagram: @MissSashaDeol
Facebook: www.facebook.com/the7pillars

Appendix A

Fruit or Vegetable	How Many to Eat	Notes
Apple	1 small	~3 inches in diameter
Baby carrots	12	
Banana	1 large	~8 inches long
Broccoli	3 spears	~5 inches long
Celery	2 large stalks	~11-12 inches long
Cooked greens	1 cup	
Corn	1 ear	>8 inches long
Grapes	32	
Orange juice	1 cup	8 oz
Peach	1	~3 inches diameter
Plums	2 large	
Raisins	½ cup	
Raw greens	2 cups	
Red pepper	1 large	~3 inches diameter, ~4 inches long
Strawberries	8 large	
Sweet potato	1 large	2+ inches diameter
Tomato	1 large	~3 inches in diameter
Vegetable juice	1 cup	

Appendix B

How many servings should you have?[1-3]

Research on how many servings of fruits and veggies to consume daily suggests young adults, ages 19–50 years old should eat:

	Vegetables	Fruits
Men	3 cups	2 cups
Women	2 ½ cups	2 cups

*Those who exercise at least 30 minutes a day should have even more! Personally, I think 5–7 servings of fruits and veggies daily is optimal.

Appendix C

How to keep produce fresh:[1-3]

ITEM	HOW TO STORE/NOTES	NOTES
Apples	Crisper drawer	Separate any bruised/spotted apples – one bad apple will spoil the rest!
Asparagus	Fridge – cut off ½ - 1" off bottoms, place upright in a jar with 1" water in it, loosely cover exposed asparagus with plastic	
Avocados	Countertop for unripe; fridge for ripe ones	To ripen quicker, store in a paper bag at room temperature. To slow down ripening, store in the fridge
Bananas	Countertop/fruit bowl	
Bell peppers	Crisper drawer	

ITEM	HOW TO STORE/NOTES	NOTES
Broccoli	Fridge – wrap loosely in a damp kitchen towel. Do not seal in a container or plastic bag	Consume ASAP; doesn't stay fresh long
Brussels sprouts	Fridge – store them in an open container or bowl; the leaves will wilt but the inner part of the sprout will stay fresh	
Cabbage	Crisper drawer	
Carrots	Fridge – trim off green stalks, place in container of water to keep them fresh and crunchy as long as possible	
Cucumber	Crisper drawer – wrap in plastic to minimize amount of moisture and slow down the spoiling process	

ITEM	HOW TO STORE/NOTES	NOTES
Dark leafy greens	Fridge – wrap unwashed, in a damp kitchen towel and store in a plastic bag with holes	
Eggplant	Cool place away from direct sunlight at room temperature	Spoils quicker when stored in plastic
Grapes	Fridge – in a perforated plastic or paper bag	
Green beans	Crisper drawer – store unwashed, in Tupperware or a plastic bag	
Herbs	Fridge – put them in a glass of water bouquet style; trim stalks off when ready to use	
Lemons	Fridge	

ITEM	HOW TO STORE/NOTES	NOTES
Mangos	Countertop for unripe; fridge for ripe ones	To ripen quicker, store in a paper bag at room temperature. To slow down ripening, store in the fridge
Melons	Countertop until they've reached their peak then transfer them to fridge	
Mushrooms	Fridge – keep in original packaging; if they are loose, wrap them in plastic wrap with some holes poked in it	
Onions	Cool, dry place away from direct sunlight	Store away from potatoes; they may trigger onions to sprout quicker
Oranges	Fridge or countertop	
Peaches	Countertop for unripe; fridge for ripe ones	To ripen quicker, store in a paper bag at room temperature. To slow down ripening, store in the fridge

ITEM	HOW TO STORE/NOTES	NOTES
Pears	Countertop until they are soft; then transfer to fridge	
Root vegetables (garlic, potatoes, pumpkins, beets)	Place in a natural fiber or wire mesh basket at room temperature, in a cool, dry, dark place	
Tomatoes	Countertop at room temperature until they are ripe; you can preserve them in fridge but remove them 1 day before using them to reactivate the enzymes and boost the flavor	

Anything else, I usually store in the fridge and toss out using common sense after inspecting the produce for freshness or after 1–2 weeks.

Extra Storage Tips:[3]

- Ethylene is a natural gas that is released from fruits and veggies. It speeds up ripening or rotting in sensitive fruits and vegetables that are nearby.
- To make your produce last longer, store fruits and vegetables separately since fruits release more ethylene gas than vegetables (they can spoil your veggies). For example, store apples, avocados, bananas, melons, peaches, pears and tomatoes separately from ethylene-sensitive broccoli, cabbage, cauliflower, leafy greens and lettuce.
- Avoid your kale, spinach or similar leafy greens from turning yellow quickly and going limp by storing them away from apples, bananas or peaches.
- To naturally inhibit sprouting in potatoes, store them with apples. The trace amounts of ethylene will slow sprouting in potatoes.
- Do not wash produce you plan to refrigerate.
- Remove any tight bands around your produce to let it free and breathe while stored.

APPENDIX D

EWG's Clean 15 & Dirty Dozen:[1,2]

What to buy organic and what's okay to buy conventional

BUY ORGANIC	CAN BUY CONVENTIONAL
Strawberries	Avocados
Spinach	Sweet corn
Nectarines	Pineapples
Apples	Cabbage
Grapes	Onions
Peaches	Sweet peas, frozen
Cherries	Papayas
Pears	Asparagus
Tomatoes	Mangos
Celery	Eggplant
Potatoes	Honeydew melons
Sweet bell peppers	Kiwifruit
	Cantaloupe
	Cauliflower
	Broccoli

Appendix E

What's in Season?[1, 2]

Year-Round	
Amaranth	Cherry tomatoes
Apples	Chinese eggplant
Arrowroot	Coconut
Avocados	Leeks
Bananas	Lemons
Banana squash	Lettuce
Bell peppers	Mushrooms
Black radish	Olives
Bok choy	Onions
Broccolini	Papayas
Burdock root	Parsnips
Cabbage	Pearl onions
Carrots	Potatoes
Celery	Snow peas

Fall: September, October, November	
Acorn squash	Kale
Apples	Kiwifruit
Asian pears	Key limes
Bananas	Kumquats
Beets	Lemons
Bell peppers	Lettuce
Broccoli	Limes
Brussels sprouts	Mangos
Butter lettuce	Mushrooms
Butternut squash	Onions
Cabbage	Parsnips
Cactus pears	Passion fruit
Carrots	Pears
Cauliflower	Peas
Celery	Persimmons
Chinese long beans	Pineapple
Collard greens	Potatoes
Crab apples	Pomegranates
Cranberries	Pumpkins
Date plums	Quince
Daikon radishes	Radicchio
Endives	Radishes
Garlic	Raspberries
Ginger	Spinach
Grapes	Sugar apples
Green beans	Sunflower kernels
Guava	Sweet potatoes & yams
Hearts of palm	Swiss chard
Huckleberries	Turnips
Jalapeno peppers	Winter squash

Winter: December, January, February	
Apples	Limes
Avocadoes	Mandarin oranges
Bananas	Maradol papaya
Brussels sprouts	Onions
Cabbage	Oranges
Cactus Pear	Parsnips
Carrots	Passion fruit
Celery	Pears
Clementines	Persimmons
Collard greens	Pineapples
Date plums	Potatoes
Dates	Pumpkins
Grapefruit	Sweet potatoes & yams
Kale	Swiss chard
Kiwifruit	Tangerines
Leeks	Turnips
Lemons	White squash

Spring: March, April, May	
Apples	Lemons
Apricots	Lettuce
Artichokes	Limes
Asparagus	Lychee
Bananas	Mangos
Barbados cherries	Mushrooms
Broccoli	Mustard greens
Butter lettuce	Onions
Cabbage	Oranges
Cactus	Peas
Carrots	Pineapples
Celery	Purple asparagus
Chives	Radicchio
Collard greens	Radishes
Corn	Red leaf lettuce
Fava beans	Rhubarb
Fennel	Snow peas
Garlic	Spinach
Green beans	Strawberries
Honeydew melon	Swiss chard
Jackfruit	Turnips
Kale	Watercress
Kiwifruit	White asparagus

Summer: June, July, August	
Apples	Hearts of palm
Apricots	Honeydew melon
Asian pears	Jackfruit
Avocados	Jalapeno peppers
Bananas	Key limes
Barbados cherries	Lemons
Beets	Lima beans
Bell peppers	Limes
Blackberries	Loganberries
Black currants	Loquats
Blueberries	Lychee
Boysenberries	Mangos
Butter lettuce	Mulberries
Cantaloupe	Nectarines
Carrots	Okra
Cherries	Passion fruit
Chinese long beans	Peaches
Corn	Peas
Crookneck squash	Plums
Cucumbers	Radishes
Eggplants	Raspberries
Elderberries	Shallots
Endives	Strawberries
Figs	Sugar snap peas
Garlic	Summer squash
Grape tomatoes	Tomatillo
Grapefruit	Tomatoes
Grapes	Watermelon
Green beans	Yukon gold potatoes
Edamame	Zucchini

References

Pillar I: Nutrition

1. Goleman, D. (2014). *Emotional intelligence.* London: Bloomsbury Publishing.

2. Csikszentmihalyi, M. (2008). *Flow: the psychology of optimal experience.* New York: Harper Perennial Modern Classics.

3. Auvichayapat, P., Prapochanung, M., Tunkamnerdthai, O., Sripanidkulchai, B.-O., Auvichayapat, N., Thinkhamrop, B., ... Hongprapas, P. (2008). Effectiveness of green tea on weight reduction in obese Thais: A randomized, controlled trial. *Physiology & Behavior, 93*(3), 486–491. doi:10.1016/j.physbeh.2007.10.009

4. Nagao, T., Hase, T., & Tokimitsu, I. (2007). A Green Tea Extract High in Catechins Reduces Body Fat and Cardiovascular Risks in Humans*. *Obesity, 15*(6), 1473–1483. doi:10.1038/oby.2007.176

5. Westerterp-Plantenga, M. (2010). Green tea catechins, caffeine and body-weight regulation. *Physiology & Behavior, 100*(1), 42–46. doi:10.1016/j.physbeh.2010.02.005

6. Ioakimidis I, et al. (2011*). Description of Chewing and Food Intake over the Course of a Meal.* doi:10.1016/j.physbeh.2011.07.021

7. Li, J., Zhang, N., Hu, L., Li, Z., Li, R., Li, C., & Wang, S. (2011). Improvement in chewing activity reduces energy intake in one meal and modulates plasma gut hormone concentrations in obese and lean young Chinese men. *American Journal of Clinical Nutrition, 94*(3), 709–716. doi:10.3945/ajcn.111.015164

8. Stevens, J. H. (2011). *Eating and Swallowing Guidelines.* Retrieved September 1, 2019, from

https://www.dshs.wa.gov/sites/default/files/DDA/dd
a/documents/Eating Swallowing Guidelines.pdf

9. Cirino, E. (2019, January 22). *How Many Times
    Should You Chew Your Food?* Retrieved June 30,
    2019, from https://www.healthline.com/health/how-
    many-times-should-you-chew-your-food

10. Cassady BA, et al. (2009). *Mastication of Almonds:
    Effects of Lipid Bioaccessibility, Appetite, and Hormone
    Response.* doi:10.3945/ajcn.2008.26669

11. Higgs S, et al. (2013). *Prolonged Chewing at Lunch
    Decreases Later Snack Intake.*
    doi:10.1016/j.appet.2012.11.019

12. Cirino, E., & Biggers, A. (2018, October 17). *How Many
    Times Should You Chew Your Food?* Retrieved
    September 5, 2019, from https://www.healthline.com/
    health/how-many-times-should-you-chew-your-food.

13. O'Reilly, G. A., Cook, L., Spruijt-Metz, D., & Black, D.
    S. (2014). Mindfulness-based interventions for obesity-
    related eating behaviours: a literature review. *Obesity
    reviews : an official journal of the International
    Association for the Study of Obesity, 15*(6), 453–461.
    doi:10.1111/obr.12156

14. Robinson, E., Aveyard, P., Daley, A., Jolly, K., Lewis, A.,
    Lycett, D., & Higgs, S. (2013). Eating attentively: a
    systematic review and meta-analysis of the effect of
    food intake memory and awareness on eating. *The
    American journal of clinical nutrition, 97*(4), 728–742.
    doi:10.3945/ajcn.112.045245

15. Aller, E. E., Abete, I., Astrup, A., Martinez, J. A., & van
    Baak, M. A. (2011). Starches, sugars and obesity.
    Nutrients, 3(3), 341–369. doi:10.3390/nu3030341

16. Geliebter, A., Grillot, C. L., Aviram-Friedman, R., Haq,
    S., Yahav, E., & Hashim, S. A. (2015). Effects of
    Oatmeal and Corn Flakes Cereal Breakfasts on Satiety,
    Gastric Emptying, Glucose, and Appetite-Related

Hormones. *Annals of Nutrition and Metabolism*, *66*(2-3), 93–103. doi: 10.1159/000365933

17. Chandler-Laney, P. C., Morrison, S. A., Goree, L. L., Ellis, A. C., Casazza, K., Desmond, R., & Gower, B. A. (2014). Return of hunger following a relatively high carbohydrate breakfast is associated with earlier recorded glucose peak and nadir. *Appetite*, *80*, 236–241. doi:10.1016/j.appet.2014.04.031

18. George A. Bray, MD; Steven R. Smith, MD; et al Leanne M. Redman, PhD. "Effect of Dietary Protein Content on Weight Gain, Energy Expenditure, and Body Composition During Overeating." *Journal of the American Medical Association* 2012;307(1):47-55. doi:10.1001/jama.2011.1918

19. La Bounty, P. M., Campbell, B. I., Wilson, J., Galvan, E., Berardi, J., Kleiner, S. M., ... Antonio, J. (2011). International Society of Sports Nutrition position stand: meal frequency. *Journal of the International Society of Sports Nutrition*, *8*, 4. doi:10.1186/1550-2783-8-4

20. Smeets, A. J., & Westerterp-Plantenga, M. S. (2008). Acute effects on metabolism and appetite profile of one meal difference in the lower range of meal frequency. *British Journal of Nutrition*, *99*(6), 1316–1321. doi:10.1017/s0007114507877646

21. Ellison, B., Lusk, J. L., & Davis, D. (2013). Looking at the label and beyond: the effects of calorie labels, health consciousness, and demographics on caloric intake in restaurants. *The international journal of behavioral nutrition and physical activity*, *10*, 21. doi:10.1186/1479-5868-10-21

22. Herman, C. P. (2015). The social facilitation of eating. A review. *Appetite*, *86*, 61–73. doi:10.1016/j.appet.2014.09.016

23. Sominsky, L., & Spencer, S. J. (2014). Eating behavior and stress: a pathway to obesity. *Frontiers in psychology, 5,* 434. doi:10.3389/fpsyg.2014.00434

24. Caton, S., Bate, L., & Hetherington, M. (2007). Acute effects of an alcoholic drink on food intake: Aperitif versus co-ingestion. *Physiology & Behavior, 90*(2-3), 368–375. doi:10.1016/j.physbeh.2006.09.028

25. Caton, S. J., Nolan, L. J., & Hetherington, M. M. (2015). Alcohol, Appetite and Loss of Restraint. *Current Obesity Reports, 4*(1), 99–105. doi:10.1007/s13679-014-0130-y

26. Harvard Health Publishing. (2018, May). *When it comes to protein, how much is too much?* Retrieved August 18, 2019, from https://www.health.harvard.edu/diet-and-weight-loss/when-it-comes-to-protein-how-much-is-too-much

27. Panel on Macronutrients, Panel on the Definition of Dietary Fiber, Subcommittee on Upper Reference Levels of Nutrients, Subcommittee on Interpretation and Uses of Dietary Reference Intakes, and the Standing Committee on the Scientific Evaluation of Dietary Reference Intakes, Food and Nutrition Board, Institute of Medicine of the National Academies. Dietary Reference Intakes for Energy, Carbohydrate, Fiber, Fat, Fatty Acids, Cholesterol, Protein, and Amino Acids [Internet]. Washington, DC: National Academies Press; 2005 [cited 2019 Mar 17]. Available from: http://www.nap.edu/catalog.php?record_id=10490

28. Russell J de Souza, George A Bray, et al "Effects of 4 weight-loss diets differing in fat, protein, and carbohydrate on fat mass, lean mass, visceral adipose tissue, and hepatic fat: results from the POUNDS LOST trial." *American Journal of Clinical Nutrition* January 18, 2012. doi:10.4016/39369.01

29. Gunnars, K. (2018, July 05). Protein Intake – How Much Protein Should You Eat Per Day? Retrieved

August 16, 2019, from https://www.healthline.com/nutrition/how-much-protein-per-day

30. Ortinau, L. C., Hoertel, H. A., Douglas, S. M., & Leidy, H. J. (2014). Effects of high-protein vs. high- fat snacks on appetite control, satiety, and eating initiation in healthy women. *Nutrition journal, 13,* 97. doi:10.1186/1475-2891-13-97

31. Esselstyn, C. B. (2011). *Prevent and reverse heart disease: The revolutionary, scientifically proven, nutrition-based cure.* New York: Avery.

32. Esselstyn, C. (2019). Dr. Esselstyn's Prevent & Reverse Heart Disease Program: Make yourself heart attack proof. Retrieved July 7, 2019, from http://www.dresselstyn.com/site/

33. Esselstyn, C. (2019). FAQ: Dr. Esselstyn's Prevent & Reverse Heart Disease Program. Retrieved June 30, 2019, from https://www.dresselstyn.com/site/faq/

34. USDA. (2019). Choose MyPlate. Retrieved June 23, 2019, from https://www.choosemyplate.gov/

35. USDA. (2019, July 18). All About the Fruit Group. Retrieved August 1, 2019, from https://www.choosemyplate.gov/fruit

36. USDA. (2019, July 18). All about the Vegetable Group. Retrieved August 16, 2019, from https://www.choosemyplate.gov/vegetables

37. Chang T, et al. (2012). *Inadequate Hydration, BMI, and Obesity Among Us Adults.* doi:*10.1370/afm.1951*

38. Familydoctor.org. (2019, June 13). Dehydration. Retrieved July 7, 2019, from https://familydoctor.org/dehydration/

39. Palsdottir, H. (2016, November 08). Drink 8 Glasses of Water a Day: Fact or Fiction? Retrieved May 3, 2019, from https://www.healthline.com/nutrition/8-glasses-of-water-per-day

40. USGS. (2019). The Water in You. Retrieved August 23, 2019, from https://www.usgs.gov/special-topic/water-science-school/science/water-you-water-and-human-body

41. Iftikhar, N. (2018, September 28). How to Tell If You're Dehydrated: Signs, Skin Test, in Pregnancy, More. Retrieved July 7, 2019, from https://www.healthline.com/health/how-to-tell-if-youre-dehydrated

42. Hopkins Medicine. (n.d.). Constipation. Retrieved June 3, 2019, from https://www.hopkinsmedicine.org/health/conditions-and-diseases/constipation

43. Mayo Clinic. (2017, October 27). Urine Color. Retrieved July 23, 2019, from https://www.mayoclinic.org/diseases-conditions/urine-color/symptoms-causes/syc-20367333

44. Meyers, C. G. (2019). Which Plants Provide Vitamin B-12? Retrieved August 23, 2019, from https://www.livestrong.com/article/449142-what-plants-provide-vitamin-b12/

45. Greger, M. (2017). *How not to die.* Place of publication not identified: Pan Books.

Pillar II: Social

1. Berkman, L. F., & Syme, S. L. (1979). Social Networks, Host Resistance, And Mortality: A Nine-Year Follow-Up Study of Alameda County Residents. *American Journal of Epidemiology, 109*(2), 186–204. doi:10.1093/oxfordjournals.aje.a112674

2. Brummett, B. H., Barefoot, J. C., Siegler, I. C., Clapp-Channing, N. E., Lytle, B. L., Bosworth, H. B., … Mark, D. B. (2001). Characteristics of Socially Isolated Patients with Coronary Artery Disease Who Are at Elevated Risk for Mortality. *Psychosomatic Medicine, 63*(2), 267–272. doi:10.1097/00006842-200103000-00010

3. Everson-Rose, S. A., & Lewis, T. T. (2005). Psychosocial Factors and Cardiovascular Diseases. *Annual Review of Public Health, 26*(1), 469–500. doi: 10.1146/annurev.publhealth.26.021304.144542

4. Hughes, M. E., & Waite, L. J. (2009). Marital Biography and Health at Mid-Life. *Journal of Health and Social Behavior, 50*(3), 344–358. doi:10.1177/002214650905000307

5. Reblin, M., & Uchino, B. N. (2008). Social and emotional support and its implication for health. *Current Opinion in Psychiatry, 21*(2), 201–205. doi:10.1097/yco.0b013e3282f3ad89

6. Uchino, B. N. (2006). Social Support and Health: A Review of Physiological Processes Potentially Underlying Links to Disease Outcomes. *Journal of Behavioral Medicine, 29*(4), 377–387. doi:10.1007/s10865-006-9056-5

7. Umberson, D., & Montez, J. K. (2010). Social Relationships and Health: A Flashpoint for Health Policy. *Journal of Health and Social Behavior, 51*(1_suppl). doi:10.1177/0022146510383501

8. Luna, A. (2019, May 29). 6 Types of Energy Vampires That Emotionally Exhaust You. Retrieved September 11, 2019, from https://lonerwolf.com/types-energy-vampire/.

Pillar III: Emotional

1. Diener, E., & Chan, M. Y. (2011). Happy People Live Longer: Subjective Well-Being Contributes to Health and Longevity. *Applied Psychology: Health and Well-Being, 3*(1), 1–43. doi:10.1111/j.1758-0854.2010.01045.x

2. Hamilton, D. (2019). *Little Book of Kindness*. Place of publication not identified: GAIA Books LTD.

3. PowerofPositivity. (2019, August 27). 24 Affirmations To Help You Build Positive Self-Talk. Retrieved September 27, 2019, from https://www.powerofpositivity.com/24-affirmations-help-build-positive-self-talk/.

4. Holland, K., & Legg, T. J. (2018, October 17). Positive Self-Talk: How Talking to Yourself Is a Good Thing. Retrieved September 27, 2019, from https://www.healthline.com/health/positive-self-talk#benefits-of-self--talk.

Pillar IV: Mental

1. Whitbourne, S. K., Dr. (2017, May 13). 5 Reasons to Clear the Clutter out of Your Life. Retrieved February 9, 2019, from https://www.psychologytoday.com/us/blog/fulfillment-any-age/201705/5-reasons-clear-the-clutter-out-your-life

2. Roster, C. A., Ferrari, J. R., & Jurkat, M. P. (2016). The dark side of home: Assessing possession 'clutter' on subjective well-being. *Journal of Environmental Psychology,* 4632-41. doi:10.1016/j.jenvp.2016.03.003

3. Vartanian, L. R., Kernan, K. M., & Wansink, B. (2017). Clutter, chaos, and overconsumption: The role of mind-set in stressful and chaotic food environments. *Environment and Behavior, 49*(2), 215-223. doi:10.1177/0013916516628178

4. Bliese, P. D., Edwards, J. R., & Sonnentag, S. (2017). Stress and well-being at work: A century of empirical trends reflecting theoretical and societal influences. *Journal of Applied Psychology, 102*(3), 389-402. doi:10.1037/apl0000109

5. Cutting, J. E., & Armstrong, K. L. (2016). Facial expression, size, and clutter: Inferences from movie structure to emotion judgments and back. *Attention,*

Perception, & Psychophysics, 78(3), 891-901.
doi:10.3758/s13414-015-1003-5

6. Amer, T., Campbell, K. L., & Hasher, L. (2016). Cognitive control as a double-edged sword. *Trends in Cognitive Sciences, 20*(12), 905-915. doi:10.1016/j.tics.2016.10.002

7. Moran, A., Guillot, A., Macintyre, T., & Collet, C. (2011). Re-imagining motor imagery: Building bridges between cognitive neuroscience and sport psychology. *British Journal of Psychology*, 103(2), 224–247. doi:10.1111/j.2044-8295.2011.02068.

8. Ridderinkhof, K. R., & Brass, M. (2015). How Kinesthetic Motor Imagery works: A predictive-processing theory of visualization in sports and motor expertise. *Journal of Physiology-Paris, 109*(1-3), 53–63. doi:10.1016/j.jphysparis.2015.02.003

9. Bregman, P. (2014, July 23). How (and Why) to Stop Multitasking. Retrieved from https://hbr.org/2010/05/how-and-why-to-stop-multitaski.html

10. Craven, C. (2018, October 7). Multiple Sclerosis and Multitasking. Retrieved from https://www.healthline.com/health-news/talking-while-walking-can-be-difficult-for-people-with-ms

11. Pivoriunaite, L. (2016, November 14). Multitasking is Failing: How to Stay Connected. Retrieved from https://www.lifehack.org/494988/multitasking-is-failing-how-to-stay-connected

12. Rock, D. (2009, October 4). Easily Distracted? Retrieved from https://www.psychologytoday.com/intl/blog/your-brain-work/200910/easily-distracted

13. Anderson, J. A., Dalton, E. R., & Basker, M. A. (1979). Insomnia and hypnotherapy. *Journal of the Royal Society of Medicine, 72*(10), 734–739.

14. Jensen, M. P., Jamieson, G. A., Lutz, A., Mazzoni, G., McGeown, W. J., Santarcangelo, E. L., … Terhune, D.

B. (2017). New directions in hypnosis research: strategies for advancing the cognitive and clinical neuroscience of hypnosis. *Neuroscience of consciousness*, *3*(1), nix004. doi:10.1093/nc/nix004

15. Mayo Clinic Staff. (2018, November 1). Hypnosis. Retrieved from https://www.mayoclinic.org/tests-procedures/hypnosis/about/pac-20394405

16. Stanford Medicine. (2016, July 28). Study identifies brain areas altered during hypnotic trances. Retrieved from https://med.stanford.edu/news/all-news/2016/07/study-identifies-brain-areas-altered-during-hypnotic-trances.html

17. Zimberoff, D. (2018, March 22). What Is the Difference Between Hypnosis and Hypnotherapy? How does hypnotherapy work? Retrieved from https://web.wellness-institute.org/blog/bid/256330/What-Is-the-Difference-Between-Hypnosis-and-Hypnotherapy

18. Gladwell, Malcolm. *Blink: the Power of Thinking without Thinking*. CNIB, 2006.

Pillar V: Spiritual

1. Goyal, M., Singh, S., Sibinga, E., Gould, N., Rowland-Seymour, A., Sharma, R., … Cramer, H. (2014). Meditation Programs for Psychological Stress and Well-being: A Systematic Review and Meta-analysis. *Deutsche Zeitschrift Für Akupunktur*, *57*(3), 26–27. doi:10.1016/j.dza.2014.07.007

2. Rosenkranz, M. A., Davidson, R. J., Maccoon, D. G., Sheridan, J. F., Kalin, N. H., & Lutz, A. (2013). A comparison of mindfulness-based stress reduction and an active control in modulation of neurogenic inflammation. *Brain, Behavior, and Immunity*, *27*, 174–184. doi:10.1016/j.bbi.2012.10.013

3. Orme-Johnson, D. W., & Barnes, V. A. (2014). Effects of the Transcendental Meditation Technique on Trait Anxiety: A Meta-Analysis of Randomized Controlled Trials. *The Journal of Alternative and Complementary Medicine*, *20*(5), 330–341. doi:10.1089/acm.2013.0204

4. Thrope, M. (2017, June 5). 12 Science-Based Benefits of Meditation. Retrieved November 1, 2019, from https://www.healthline.com/nutrition/12-benefits-of-meditation.

5. White, M. P., Alcock, I., Grellier, J., Wheeler, B. W., Hartig, T., Warber, S. L., … Fleming, L. E. (2019). Spending at least 120 minutes a week in nature is associated with good health and wellbeing. *Scientific Reports*, *9*(1). doi:10.1038/s41598-019-44097-3

6. Barton, J., & Pretty, J. (2010). What is the Best Dose of Nature and Green Exercise for Improving Mental Health? A Multi-Study Analysis. *Environmental Science & Technology*, *44*(10), 3947–3955. doi:10.1021/es903183r

7. Weatherford, D. (n.d.). Slow Dance. Retrieved October 3, 2019, from http://www.davidlweatherford.com/slowdance.html.

Pillar VI: Physical

1. Examining Gym Cleanliness. (n.d.). Retrieved June 7, 2019, from https://www.fitrated.com/resources/examining-gym-cleanliness/.

2. Semeco, A. (2018, May 31). Pre-Workout Nutrition: What to Eat Before a Workout. Retrieved July 31, 2019, from https://www.healthline.com/nutrition/eat-before-workout.

3. Aragon, A., & Schoenfeld, B. (2013). Nutrient Timing Revisited. *Functional Foods*, 65–89. doi:10.1201/b16307-5

4. Hawley, J. A., & Burke, L. M. (1997). Effect of meal frequency and timing on physical performance. *British Journal of Nutrition, 77*(S1). doi:10.1079/bjn19970107

5. Aragon, A., & Schoenfeld, B. (2013). Nutrient Timing Revisited. *Functional Foods*, 65–89. doi:10.1201/b16307-5

6. Greger, M. (2017). *How not to die.* Place of publication not identified: Pan Books.

7. Bubnis, D. (2018, July 20). 8 Foam Rolling Moves. Retrieved June 15, 2019, from https://www.healthline.com/health/fitness-exercise/foam-rolling-how-to#1.

Pillar VII: Integrity

1. Kerr, J. M. (2016, May 20). Four principles for high integrity. Retrieved September 13, 2019, from https://www.management-issues.com/opinion/7178/four-principles-for-high-integrity/.

Appendix A

1. Lehman, S. (2019, July 23). Serving Sizes for 18 Fruits and Vegetables. Retrieved August 16, 2019, from https://www.verywellfit.com/serving-sizes-for-18-fruits-and-vegetables-2506865

Appendix B

1. Bere E, Brug J, Klepp KI. Why Do Boys Eat Less Fruit and Vegetables Than Girls? Public Health Nutr. 2008;11(3):321-5. doi:10.1017/S1368980007000729

2. Bere E, Brug J, Klepp KI. Why Do Boys Eat Less Fruit and Vegetables Than Girls? Public Health Nutr. 2008;11(3):321-5. doi:10.1017/S1368980007000729

3. Lehman, S. (2019, June 24). How Many Cups of Vegetables Do You Need per Day? Retrieved August 23,

2019, from https://www.verywellfit.com/recommended-vegetable-servings-per-day-by-age-2506868

Appendix C

1. 8fit.com. (2019). How to Store Fruits and Vegetables to Preserve Freshness. Retrieved August 1, 2019, from https://8fit.com/nutrition/how-to-store-fruits-vegetables-for-freshness/
2. Bob Mueller, Using Ethylne, Potato Grower Magazine, August 2013 Issue Published online: Aug 04, 2013.
3. Editors, V. T. (2007, June 21). Spoiled Rotten - How to Store Fruits and Vegetables. Retrieved September 2, 2019, from http://www.vegetariantimes.com/article/spoiled-rotten-how-to-store-fruits-and-vegetables/

Appendix D

1. Environmental Working Group. (2019). Clean Fifteen™ Conventional Produce with the Least Pesticides. Retrieved June 14, 2019, from https://www.ewg.org/foodnews/clean-fifteen.php
2. Environmental Working Group. (2019). Dirty Dozen™ Fruits and Vegetables with the Most Pesticides. Retrieved June 14, 2019, from https://www.ewg.org/foodnews/dirty-dozen.php

Appendix E

1. Fruitsandveggies.com. (2019). What Fruits & Vegetables are in Season? Retrieved August 16, 2019, from https://fruitsandveggies.org/stories/what-fruits-and-vegetables-are-in-season/
2. USDA. (2019). Seasonal Produce Guide. Retrieved September 1, 2019, from https://snaped.fns.usda.gov/seasonal-produce-guide

Made in the USA
Monee, IL
09 December 2022

20487140R00066